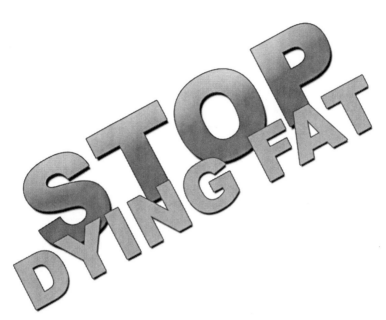

AUG 13
CH

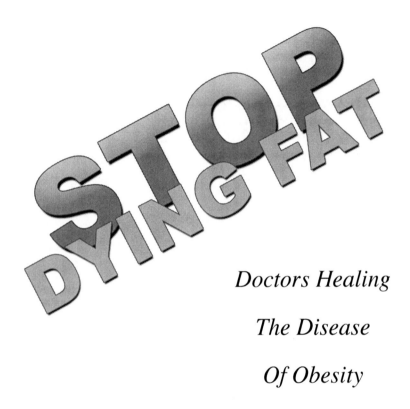

STOP DYING FAT

Doctors Healing

The Disease

Of Obesity

ELEAZAR M. KADILE MD

Director, *Center for Integrative Medicine*

Home of the **KadileAtric Power Principle®** and
the **Slendergenic Meal Plan**

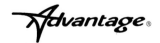

Published by Advantage, Charleston, South Carolina.
Member of Advantage Media Group.

ADVANTAGE is a registered trademark and the Advantage colophon is a trademark of Advantage Media Group, Inc.

Printed in the United States of America.

ISBN: 978-1-59932-190-5
LCCN: 2012953108

This publication is designed to provide accurate and authoritative information in regard to the subject matter covered. It is sold with the understanding that the publisher is not engaged in rendering legal, accounting, or other professional services. If legal advice or other expert assistance is required, the services of a competent professional person should be sought.

Advantage Media Group is proud to be a part of the Tree Neutral® program. Tree Neutral offsets the number of trees consumed in the production and printing of this book by taking proactive steps such as planting trees in direct proportion to the number of trees used to print books. To learn more about Tree Neutral, please visit www.treeneutral.com. To learn more about Advantage's commitment to being a responsible steward of the environment, please visit www.advantagefamily.com/green

Advantage Media Group is a leading publisher of business, motivation, and self-help authors. Do you have a manuscript or book idea that you would like to have considered for publication? Please visit www.advantagefamily.com or call 1.866.775.1696

To KRISTIAN ELEAZAR KADILE, d. 1995

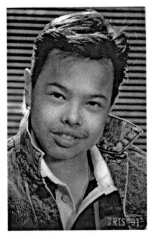

Your time with us was too brief. We could not save your life, but the challenges you faced inspired us to question standard medical practices and find new ways to help those who lost hope. As a result, many lives have been changed, many lives have been saved. Your brief life continues to save lives.

After all these years, Son, our love still grows.

To GENIA ILECKI KADILE, d. 2012

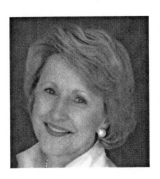

My wife, my companion, my caregiver, the mother of my children and the inspiration for my work, my soul mate, you have been the all-too-often unspoken wisdom behind all that I have done in medicine and in my life. You created a space for me to grow as a man and as a physician. You held our children in love and safety, held them through long and agonizing nights of fear and worry. You were the rock of all of our lives and now that you have passed on to your "next adventure," we own your love of us as our greatest treasure. Even beyond the grave, you teach and guide us. Thank you for taking such good care of us all.

—Eleazar

Life is like holding a butterfly.

If you hold it too tightly, you'll crush it to death.

If you hold it too loosely, it will fly away.

Hold it just right—gently, tenderly, and lovingly—it will be with you.

—Chinese proverb

TABLE OF CONTENTS

DISCLAIMER

The **KadileAtric Power Principle®** is not appropriate for anyone with untreated ovarian failure—namely, cyst, cancer, endometriosis; untreated thyroid disorder; untreated adrenal failure; or gout predisposition, because the foundation of KPP involves hormonal balancing, nutritional support, digestive enzymes, and a high-protein diet. These untreated medical conditions could be aggravated.

A medical practice is not an exact science; it is more of an art. The inadvertent use of hyperbole in this text should be taken with a grain of salt. As always, medical outcomes are not typical and may vary from individual to individual, and the KadileAtric Power Principle® is not an exception.

The information in this book is based solely on Dr. Kadile's opinions and is presented for general informational purposes only. It is not intended to replace a one-on-one relationship with a qualified health-care professional and is not intended as medical diagnosis or advice.

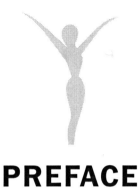

PREFACE

Those who trust chance must abide by the results of chance. They have no legitimate complaint against anyone but themselves.
—Calvin Coolidge

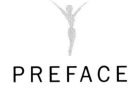

PREFACE

I wrote this book for you. I wrote it to inspire you to take what could be the most important step of your life, a step toward health, happiness, well-being, and an outlook on life that you may have long ago given up achieving. I wrote it for people who are suffering from the disease of obesity, AND who are looking for a medically sound, physician-supervised treatment for their disease. This is a book for patients who want to do what it takes to lose weight and be healthy again. Throughout this book you will be reading real-life stories from real-life people who have changed their lives because of the **Kadile-Atric Power Principle®**. Their testimonies, by far, will be the most inspirational part of the text. They are the flesh and blood testimonies that will inspire you to have the life you want.

This book lays out a set of medical and personal protocols that I call the **KadileAtric Power Principle®** (KPP) and **Slendergenic** foods, which are the basis for what I believe can be the treatment for the disease of obesity in the chronically overweight or obese person. These protocols must be supervised by a physician or licensed medical professional who has the breadth and depth of knowledge to understand how KPP works and has quick access to the diagnostic tools needed to implement KPP.

Physicians and medical providers who have been authorized by me to use the KadileAtric Power Principle® and Slendergenic meal plans are fully versed in the subtle yet powerful protocols that first identify key imbalances and obstructive factors that prevent patients from losing weight. Then, when the bodily systems are balanced, affect rapid weight-loss without surgery, synthetic drugs, or exercise. This four-part set of protocols not only causes patients to experience dramatic controlled weight loss, but may also significantly remit or heal other diseases that accompany excess weight.

This program requires substantive changes in the way obese people live and experience their bodies. **It is an easy program** to follow because all of its details are laid out in black and white. KPP patients must know exactly what's going on in every part of the program. That is essential. Also, it is easy because it is effective. It works; patients lose significant amounts of weight quickly without exercise, surgery, drugs, or exotic foods. It is easy because in KPP patients feel empowered, respected, supported, and encouraged to take control of their health in ways that they may not have experienced in the past. KPP is easy because the patient's physician partner will always be there to answer questions and help figure out the best way to lose weight and stay healthy.

KPP could be perceived as **a difficult program** because it requires that patients learn how to **enjoy change,** to study how they are changing, and become fascinated with the amazing things a body can do as it changes. KPP patients know that the most basic change comes from no longer being disabled by their weight. This is a change that comes at the price of having to think differently, act, and eat differently, relate to their doctor differently, and be in relationships with family, friends, and community differently because, without the disease of obesity, they are different people. Losing weight, like staying sober for the drug addict, requires vigilance, concentration, honesty, perseverance, and a degree of humility. A sense of humor helps a great deal too. These are the factors that can make the Kadile-Atric Power Principle® difficult—and exciting.

As you read this book, if you want to get a more detailed view of the KPP protocols (four parts), please turn to Chapter Five. There they are presented in some detail. You will get a sense of how the protocols unfold and develop. However, let me warn you, dear patient, at the very start, that KPP is not a fill-in-the-blanks program, where you simply follow the doctor's orders and get the cure. KPP, as you will learn throughout this book, will require that you become involved, take charge, learn many new things, and commit yourself to being supported by your doctor and medical staff in becoming a healthy person. This is not a one-size-fits-all program. Every patient is different, which means that all patients must be far more involved in their ongoing recovery from the disease of obesity in order to sustain the success they hoped for when they started KPP. Each chapter in this book will give you both a new perspective on how you can become healthy, and on the new challenges that you face when you become involved in that process.

Now it's up to you to evaluate the balance between easy and difficult and whether you feel ready to find a physician or medical provider trained in the KadileAtric Power Principle® to help you heal the disease of obesity. You will be a different person for it. Your life, like your body, may be totally unrecognizable to those people who have only known you as overweight. You may have to reintroduce yourself to them, and to yourself. Your life can change that dramatically. I want KPP to be there to help you.

If you need help finding a physician I have trained and authorized to use the KadileAtric Power Principle®, please do not hesitate to contact me at:

The Center for Integrative Medicine
1538 Bellevue Street
Green Bay, Wisconsin 54311
(920) 468-9442
www.KPPMD.com

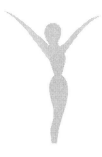

ONE

INTRODUCTION

No matter how hard you work for success, if your thought

is saturated with the fear of failure, it will kill your efforts,

neutralize your endeavors, and make success impossible.

—Charles Baudouin

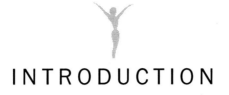

INTRODUCTION

TRUTH BE TOLD

As you begin reading this book, let me make several things perfectly clear.

First, I will always tell you the truth about obesity, about weight and the power it can have over your life, about the complex (and beautiful) web of interdependent systems that contribute to health and wellness (and disease and dysfunction), and about the limits of how the things I know about the disease of obesity might be helpful to you.

Second, if you have the disease of obesity, I will always respect and honor your humanity, your feelings, your opinions, your strengths, and your weaknesses. You are a human being just like me, deserving of love, respect, attention, help, and support.

Third, I will not blame you for having the disease of obesity. **It's not your fault.** There are many factors that contribute to the disease we call obesity. Many, if not most of them, are *not* due to a lack of willpower or self-control on your part, or some character flaw that you have not adequately addressed. The path to healing the disease of obesity will require many changes in your behaviors, but your current behaviors are not the sole cause of your obesity.

Obesity is caused by complex imbalances both within the patient and the patient's environment. Some imbalances are exacerbated by poor dietary choices based on bad dietary information, personal history, and psychological patterns. Together, the physiological, psychological, social, and environmental causes of the disease of obesity create a vortex into which you, the patient, might feel drawn into and unable to get out of.

The role of the physician in healing this disease is to do sufficient research into each of these factors, study how these factors interrelate, find noninvasive remedies to alleviate each factor, and then support patients in making changes in their personal habits that will allow them to lose weight, regain health, and take charge of their ongoing healing. Most importantly, the role of the physician in your healing is to teach you how to stay healthy and at an appropriate weight by understanding all of the above, and teaching you to monitor your health and weight in the years ahead. A good physician will help you stay in charge of your own research into your health, and make good healthy decisions every day, every moment.

The KadileAtric Power Principle® protocols were developed to help you heal the disease of obesity. These principles are based on good science and good medicine, albeit often unconventional medicine. It is unconventional not because there is no proof that it works but because it works in ways that traditional and established medical practice has not seen fit to explore. While traditional and standard medical practice has evolved a set of approaches and protocols, these approaches tend to rule out looking at chronic medical conditions in new ways. Often, traditional medicine will celebrate what it describes as a success when all it has addressed are the symptoms of an underlying set of causes or diseases. Often doctors have tolerated side effects of medications that address symptoms when, in fact, they have not cured the disease. The KadileAtric Power Principle® is based on the core belief that the body is designed to heal itself when various bodily systems are in balance, when these systems have the natural resources that they need to function well, and that masking symptoms does not constitute a cure.

STOP DYING FAT

So, now it is time for me to say it loud and clear: I want you to **STOP DYING FAT!** And if you are like most of my patients, you want to stop dying fat too. In fact, like most of my patients, you have worked harder than your friends or family realize to lose weight, to feel better, to stop being a burden to those around you and yourself, to feel normal, to look good, to not be embarrassed by your weight and the burdens it places on your life. You want to stop being fat, and you know that the disease of obesity is killing you.

Pure and simple, you are sick and tired of going on diets promoted by beautiful people, all promising amazing results and a great love life, and each and every one of these diets wants you to believe that if you just changed what you ate, you'd be beautiful too. Well, my friend, that just isn't so. What and how you eat is only a part of why you have the disease of obesity, and I want to help you. I want you to live a long and healthy life. I want you to know subtle levels of well-being that bring you to a new consciousness of what life can be like, a life without the burdens that excess weight and its accompanying diseases can place on you.

So, what is it going to take for you to stop dying fat and start living a new healthy life?

First, it's going to take **good information** about your condition, information that will be generated by your doctor from an array of very sophisticated, noninvasive tests that tell what is going on in your body, in every system in your body. Very important information will come from you as you share many things with your doctor about your life, how you feel when you're feeling poorly, what your habits are, what kind of support you have for changing your life, and so forth. At this point, you will see that you are in a 50/50 partnership with your doctor, both of you contracting to do research into your health, advising each other on what works and what doesn't work, studying how the pieces of your life mount up to create a tsunami of illness or a mountain of health.

Second, it's going to take **motivation to change** many things about how you live your life, how you understand what constitutes a good life for you, how you make choices and why. You will focus on those aspects that motivate you the most so that you can utilize the energy of that motivation to help you change, and, as you will see later in this book, your motivation to "stop dying fat" will change as you start reaching some of the weight-loss goals that you never thought were possible. The things that motivate you to start this medical protocol we call the KadileAtric Power Principle® will most likely not be the things that motivate you to stay healthy in the future. Motivation changes as you find yourself higher on the mountain of health. Change is both exciting and difficult. Change is exciting because it represents a moment toward your goals of health and well-being. Change is difficult because it requires you to take risks, try new behaviors, and experience life in different ways, looking at yourself in a new light, and then living that change in front of your family, friends, colleagues, and community. Yes, change is both exciting and difficult.

Third, in order to stop dying fat, you will have to **learn a lot.** You will be going "back to school" to learn how the basic science of life, the science of your body, works (or how it doesn't work), and how to apply what you know to how you act. You will need to become the foremost expert on your own health, the primary researcher into the amazing collection of interdependent systems that make up your body. You will study how your mind helps or hinders how your body is experienced by you. You will study the social systems that change as you change. You may even learn how to cook and eat in new and exciting ways. Some may experience new aspects of their spiritual lives as they experience profound changes in their relationship with their new and healthy bodies. You will learn how to communicate what you know to people who can help you so that you will get the best advice, support, and medical treatment possible from the professionals who will accompany you on your continuing journey toward health. You will learn that you are strong, intelligent, clear, dedicated, fragile, fallible, and funny. You will learn a lot about yourself, and very possibly find that you know yourself, really know yourself, for the first time.

And finally, you will have to be **vigilant and extremely honest** in your quest to stop dying fat. The protocols that you will be learning in this book require that you develop a keen awareness of when you are fooling yourself, when you are strong or weak, when you are honest or truthful. As in any recovery program, vigilance and honesty are the fundamental virtues that support the change that you desire. Some people need the help of those family members, friends, and professionals they trust in order to achieve levels of honesty that profound change requires. Some people manage to do it on their own, but however they do it, they will need to be able to look in the mirror and speak the truth to themselves. Now, many people find it easy to speak the truth about their flaws and failures. It is equally important, if not more important, to speak the truth to yourself about your goodness and virtues. You will need to be able to say things like: "In spite of my weaknesses, I am strong. No matter what I think I look like, I am beautiful. Regardless of the mistakes I have made in the past, I can make and dedicate myself to good and healthy choices. I am worth all the effort I am putting into being healthy. I deserve respect from myself and others. I am good."

So, you can see that I might not sound like your ordinary doctor who wants to help you lose weight. I am a doctor who is going to help you look at the whole of your life and help you put the pieces together so that you can stop dying fat. If you decide to accept the challenge to become healthy through the KPP protocols, your life will change dramatically, not only in how you look, but in how you understand who you are. You will become aware of subtleties in your life that will make your life richer, more beautiful, peaceful, and rewarding. You can see that I want the best for you in *every* way.

So, let's get started.

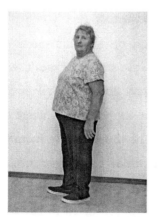

SHIRLEY MUELLER

A Life Renewed.

I couldn't go on any more, just knowing how dragged out I was, how tired I was all the time. I would watch my grandkids playing and I wasn't able to keep up with them. My gosh, I can't do anything with them. Even just walking a short distance, I'd have to say to myself, "Come on, just one more step," or walking up the stairs, I'd get out of breath, feeling like I could just keel over.

And the marvelous thing about losing this weight is that I used to have all these choking spells. We've had EMT rescue out here because I couldn't get any air, and it was only from fluids and an air pocket. It wasn't from food, but since losing the weight, I haven't had a spell. I say "Thank you, Lord." I was having them once a week, and sometimes I'd have multiple choking spells at a time. I'd have two, three of them, and my husband would get behind me and help me breath, but there wasn't anything he could do. The Heimlich maneuver didn't help. So it was either save yourself or kick the bucket, but the thing is, now, I haven't had any for a year. What if I would have one? Am I going to remember what to do now? I think that since losing weight—it has everything to do with it.

This is a funny story. When I had lost about fifty-five pounds, I went to church with my husband, Les. We're not ashamed to hold hands and be close in church. I even had my hair colored, and I had gone into church with a dress that made me look good. I bought a whole bunch of new clothes. Well, I held Les's hand in church and we left, thought nothing of it. I went to the grocery store after church by myself. As I was walking down the aisle, two elderly ladies from our church are there and one of them says rather loudly, "Well, just look at that hussy. She ought to be ashamed of herself breaking up that beautiful marriage of that nice couple. I always thought he was so dedicated to her and her to him." I look around the aisle in the grocery, wondering who in the world she's talking about. Suddenly I realized that it was me, and I said, "Who's a hussy?" and she says, "You ought to be ashamed of yourself. Les and Shirley were such a nice married couple, and you're sitting there in church holding his hand." I looked at her and said "Take a closer look at me. Who do you think I am? I'm Shirley Mueller. We've had six kids, three boys, three girls. We have five grandchildren. Remember, my daughter just adopted four? I've got three great-grandchildren." She didn't know who I was because I had lost the weight and I had my hair colored. I looked nice. She thought Les was not my husband. Embarrassed, she went off in a huff. I thought it was funny. I told Dr. Kadile that I was called a hussy.

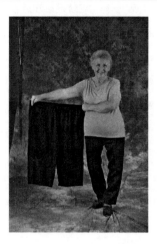

THE WEIGHT OF WEIGHT; THE POWER OF POUNDS

There is a very basic (if not somewhat cynical) law of marketing that says that if you want to sell people a product, you must first show them their pain. People usually buy things because they consciously or unconsciously believe that that new dress, tie, power tool, kitchen device, house, car, vacation—you name it—will make their life easier, happier, wiser, more peaceful, fun, etc.

If you have the disease of obesity, you are acutely aware of how your weight controls your life, and you are also acutely unaware of how many unconscious accommodations you have made to your condition.

You know, for example, that your weight is killing you. It literally weighs on you. If I were to tie a fifty-pound weight around your waist and throw you into a lake, you would know how powerful those fifty pounds are. As you sink fast, holding onto air and consciousness for as long as you can, flailing arms and legs, struggling to counteract the power of those fifty pounds, you know that that weight has power.

Yet, slowly, over time perhaps, those same 50 (or 100, or 125, or 200) pounds have been bound to your body, dragging you down in many other ways. Those pounds have controlled your wardrobe. You can only wear certain styles in order to feel comfortable or feel attractive. You usually must pay extra for those clothes. You may even have several wardrobes to accommodate the fluctuating weights that you've suffered between dieting and trying to find a normal weight. Your closets may be full of clothes you won't give away because you promise yourself that you will wear them again after the next diet. Those pounds are not only on your body but fill your closets.

Those same fifty pounds that could drag you down to the depths of the lake also keep you down on the social ladder. No one needs to tell you how "fat people" are discriminated against at work, on the street, in public transportation. There is even research that proves that many doctors and medical establishments discriminate against people with obesity, piling up mountains of fictional excuses and prejudices about why obese people are overweight. Many doctors won't treat obesity as a disease because they are convinced that "those people" are the cause of their own problem and are resistant to change. Little do these doctors realize that in many cases it is easier to cast blame than to take a different approach to the causes of their patient's condition. The problem might be that the doctor doesn't know how to help and therefore sends the patient out into the world to find answers elsewhere. Those fifty pounds have the weight of prejudice, a very heavy load indeed.

Another way of looking at the weight of weight or the power of pounds is in what is lost as a person suffers from the disease of obesity. An obese patient can oftentimes feel impotent and powerless. Having tried again and again (we know that no one works harder at losing weight than someone who suffers from obesity), obese people often feel defeated, alienated from themselves in a deeply personal way, powerless to change (because they believe that they've already tried everything), or even worse that it's not worth the effort to change because they have failed so often. Weight has the power to defeat us. It must be possible to reclaim that power, and the first step is to know how much power we've lost and how much power we can have again.

Patients with obesity also know that their weight has power over their family, community, and social networks. Excess weight controls where we can travel (and at what extra cost), how long it takes us to get there, where we can sit, and how our companions (and the anonymous traveling public) react to being near us. Eddie Murphy, the comedian in the 1996 movie, The Nutty Professor, may have tried to make obesity funny, but if you have the disease of obesity, you know for certain that it is no laughing matter. The power of pounds limits the kinds of people who may find us attractive. Excess weight is isolating, and that weight can lead to psychological weight: depression feels like a weight—and it is.

So much of the power lost through the disease of obesity can be regained. It is possible to cut the cords that bind us to those fifty pounds, lose weight, cure the disease of obesity, and stop dying fat. Yes, it is possible. I want to help you.

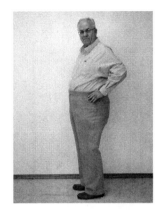

BILL SKALESKI

"I wanted a handicap sticker"

A sixty-five-year-old patient, Bill Skaleski, who lost seventy pounds in ninety-nine days, told me, "I had an impossible time trying to lose weight. It was affecting my health severely: I had high blood pressure, arthritis, and was prediabetic." He was on medications for his conditions, and his golf game, which was an important part of his life, was suffering. "I was going to ask for a handicap sticker for my car before I went on this diet because I could not walk into a store from a regular parking space anymore."

He came to me to try the KadileAtric Power Principle® program. After eighteen days, he had lost twenty-one pounds and nearly five inches from his waist. "I have not had any arthritis pain for over two weeks," he reported when he was participating in Part II of the program. "My blood pressure has been

coming in at 120/72, which would make a twenty-one-year-old envious. I have had fewer problems with my asthma, and I venture to say that the next time I take one of those insulin or prediabetic tests, I will pass with flying colors." Although his golf game hadn't improved at that point, he said he was hitting the ball about twenty yards farther.

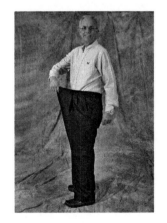

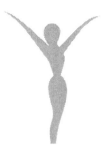

T W O

IT'S NOT YOUR FAULT YOUR FAT

The only thing in life achieved without effort is failure.

—Anonymous

IT'S NOT YOUR FAULT YOU'RE FAT

I'll bet that you never expected to hear those words coming from a medical doctor, particularly a doctor specializing in weight loss. For far too many years and in far too many ways you have heard and absorbed the message that your "weight problem" is your fault. Somehow, both blatantly and subtly, people assume that because you have the disease of obesity and are overweight, you are just not trying hard enough, don't have self-control, are impulsive, undisciplined, lazy, slothful, and unconscious of just how big you are and how bad you look. The world seems to be stacked up against you like a rigged deck of cards, and you're always the loser.

There is nothing further from the truth than the myth that "fat people" just don't try hard enough to lose weight. You know and I know for a fact that nobody tries harder to lose weight than someone who is severely overweight, someone who is obese. People suffering from the disease of obesity have probably tried every diet on the shelf, read every book, paid enormous amounts of money to buy their way to slim, and exercised harder for longer hours with very little result, and often with little to show for it but frustration, disappointment, despair, and a depleted bank account.

Few people who are not suffering from the disease of obesity understand the shame and stigma attached to being overweight. Let me list only a few in case you need to have your memory refreshed.

(Large people can sometimes be masters at suppressing the indignities they suffer in society.)

- Seats in public transportation are not designed for the comfort of the person suffering from the disease of obesity, and in order to get a seat that fits, the obese must pay first-class fare.
- There are no advertisements in newspapers and magazines that are intended to make the obese feel comfortable. All advertising models are beautifully slim and can lounge around in poses that no obese person could ever manage.
- Scientific studies demonstrate that many physicians and medical professionals do not like serving patients with obesity.
- National campaigns to combat the epidemic of obesity in this country focus primarily on food choices and exercise, two weight-loss strategies that you have already tried at great expense and effort and which have too often failed to achieve lasting or meaningful results.
- Even if the obese person can sometimes laugh at the humor of fat-people jokes, at the most intimate and subtle personal level, these jokes are never funny.
- People with the disease of obesity suffer greater risks of developing other metabolic and autoimmune related diseases.
- People with obesity have limited access to many outdoor and other recreational activities, either because of mobility issues or because size and weight restrictions make it difficult for them to manage seating restrictions.
- A study found that in one year, obese patients spent an average of $1,429 more for their medical care than did

people within a normal weight range.[1] That is a 42 percent higher cost for people who are obese.

And on and on . . . Have you had enough? Could you add a few dozen more of your own experiences to this list?

On top of the issues of shame and despair, the most debilitating side effect of the disease of obesity, is the pernicious sense that the patient with obesity is really the cause of the condition. Most patients with obesity have been led to believe that their "weight problem" is really their own fault. Many obese patients have been told that they are not trying hard enough, don't have discipline, haven't made weight loss a priority, and so forth. The litany seems endless, and at the end of the day patients with obesity simply throw up their hands and surrender to the myth that if they were "better people," they could lose weight and be welcomed back into the society of the slender and beautiful.

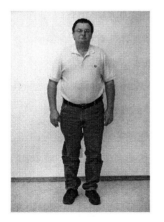

ROBERT CARROLL

People with Obesity
Suffer Discrimination

People who saw me thought I was lazy, and to tell you the truth, so did I, and also I thought that other people who were fat and fatter were lazy. I was prejudiced against fat people as well, but, boy, has that changed.

I was just with Dr. Kadile on Tuesday, and I could pick out the newcomers. I could see that they were embarrassed about their weight. I wanted to go up and give them a hug and tell them, "You're doing the right thing. I've gone through a lifestyle change, and I eat good. Yeah, I eat good. You're doing the right thing."

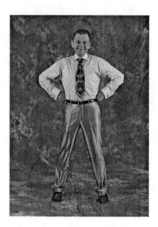

BUT THIS IS NOT THE CASE! It is not your fault that you have the disease of obesity. Let me tell you a number of reasons why. If only one or several points on the list below are true, it may be impossible for the obese patient to lose weight.

- Are metabolic functions operating optimally?
- Is the digestive system functioning well, including the presence of microscopic intestinal parasites?
- Are hormonal imbalances affecting metabolic functions, particularly thyroid and adrenal systems?
- Does the patient have food allergies?
- Are toxic metals or chemicals present in the patient and his/her environment?
- Does the patient suffer vitamin deficiencies, particularly vitamin D? Levels of essential fatty acids?
- Do medications that the obese patient takes actually prevent weight loss?

Oftentimes these complex and related medical and environmental conditions not only prevent patients from losing weight but actually cause weight gain, and still doctors often fail to recognize that when they are treating one disease, they may, in effect, be creating another: the disease of obesity.

So, let me say it again: It's not your fault that you are suffering from the disease of obesity, and should you come to a KadileAtric Power Principle® clinic. This is where we will begin to explore the ways of treating the disease of obesity from which you suffer. Our protocols look at all the ways your body functions, well or poorly, to start to put together a treatment plan that returns your body to balance and allows it to start losing weight rapidly through a medically supervised program that treats all your medical conditions in a thorough and systematic way. Once you understand why your body gains and holds onto unnecessary weight, together we can bring your body back to a balanced and normal function, and you will lose weight. It's not your fault that you have the disease of obesity. We can help you discover the causes of the disease, and step-by-step begin to help your body lose the weight that has held you prisoner for so long.

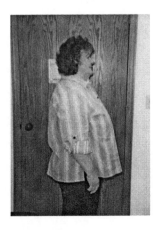

SANDY GUBBELS

Yo-Yo Dieter

Sandy Gubbels considered herself a "hard-to-lose" case. After diet upon diet had failed her, she'd given up. Sandy was born into a family of heavy women and found she was far too successful at carrying on the tradition. She thought being fat was part of her heritage. "I started gaining weight when I had children and seemed to add ten pounds with each one," Sandy recalls. "The heaviest weight I ever reached was 257 pounds."

As a wife, mother, and teacher who home-schooled her five children, Sandy thought she should have been a spokeswoman for good health. Instead, she was embarrassed about her appearance. "I certainly didn't look healthy. I could only dream of how much more I could do if I looked and felt great again. I wanted to be a walking testimonial, but I was a walking time bomb."

Sandy worked hard at losing weight. "I've been on more diets than I care to remember. I tried Atkins, the Zone Diet, a diet based on allergies, an ultrametabolism program, South Beach, and the Sonoma Diet." All this effort brought Sandy nothing but poor results. "I can lose twenty pounds on a diet," she adds, "but it always comes back, along with a few extra pounds to boot."

This wasn't her fault; the problem was that none of these methods addressed her weight problem at the core. Sandy was using conventional methods of calorie counting and exercise. These methods failed miserably because she was dealing with relentless physical hunger, cravings for sugar, salt, and fat, uncontrollable urges to eat even when she wasn't hungry, a dragging metabolism, and an unusually high amount of fat in stubborn areas such as the hips, thighs, buttocks, and waist.

Once Sandy's metabolic and hormonal imbalances were corrected, she melted off ninety-three pounds, yet she was on the low-calorie part of KPP for a surprisingly short period of time.

Sandy says her husband often comments about her weight-loss success. "He is happy that I'm now optimistic, happy, and—oh yes—romantic. He is also thrilled that I have improved my general health and well-being. I know that I look again like the girl he married, and that makes us both very happy."

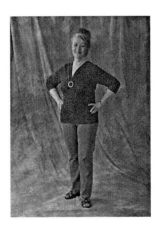

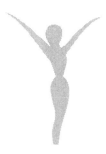

THREE

"FOOD, GLORIOUS FOOD"

Happiness is more a state of health than of wealth.

—Frank Tyger

"FOOD, GLORIOUS FOOD"

Many of you remember that great song from the hit musical *Oliver*. In it, the young Oliver Twist leads the orphans in a paean to food, all the food fantasies that they ever had pouring out, spilling over, plates, tables, and bellies full, and glorious dancing. Why? Because they didn't have any. The hunger they were suffering was satisfied in their imaginations, and their imaginations kept them going. It was a great moment of musical theater.

Many people who must lose weight feel that the only companions they will know will be hunger and want. The only way to cure the disease of obesity, for them, is to not eat, and to live in hunger and want with only the fantasy of food. The future, all too often, looks like a long, hard road of not having, endless cravings, and savage frustrations, but this is not the case with the **KadileAtric PowerPrinciple®** and the **Slendergenic meal** protocols. You will be able to eat many of your favorite foods in satisfying quantities as you begin to settle into your new weight and healthy body. This will happen because **KPP** will first address the underlying medical conditions that cause the disease of obesity to take control of your body.

THIS IS NOT A DIET PROGRAM

The **KadileAtric Power Principle®** and the **Slendergenic meal plan** together are not a diet program to lose weight. KPP and Slendergenic comprise a complementary set of medical protocols that address a real medical condition under the supervision of trained and certified physicians and medical professionals. It is not a formulaic, cookie-cutter approach to weight loss. Because the medical conditions of the person with the disease of obesity are real and profound, they are studied and treated through rigorous and sensitive medical tests and individually prescribed doses of medications and supplements, and they are regularly monitored to ensure that the underlying causes of obesity are addressed thoroughly. The final outcome is not only weight loss but a total overhaul of the patient's health and wellness, thus allowing the patient not only to potentially heal from the disease of obesity but oftentimes become free of the underlying imbalances and dysfunctions that caused many other obesity-related illnesses. So, you can clearly see KPP is not a diet program. It is much, much more.

YOUR RELATIONSHIP WITH FOOD; FOOD IS MEDICINE

Food intake and exercise have been the traditional axis upon which weight-loss programs have been built. Eat less; exercise more; lose weight. Those were the commandments in the religion of weight loss, but, if you suffer the burden of obesity, you have probably tried to obey these commandments many times with frustrating and disappointing results. So, it is important at the outset to break the frustrating cycle of intake and exercise by adjusting your relationship with food.

Through the **KPP** protocols you will learn how your body handles food, absorbs or does not absorb nutrients, how exercise might actually prevent you from losing weight at times, and when and how to eat to your satisfaction and still maintain your hard-won weight loss. So, it is important that you look at your relationship with and history of food.

Once you have started to use the KPP, you will have the opportunity to take a full and complete history of your relationship with food. You will be asked many questions about the kinds of foods you eat, when you eat them, when in your life your weight patterns began to change, and if a change in diet occurred at the same time, and so forth. You will be guided through a thorough inventory of your food and weight history before we even begin to talk about changing the foods you eat and when you eat them.

Yes, you will have to change some of the foods that you eat, and for this reason we have accompanied the KPP with the Slendergenic meal program to help you choose foods and prepare them wisely. Slendergenic recipes will guide you every step of the way as you learn to develop a new and healthy relationship to food that will bring you to your weight-loss goals and a whole new way of being.

PLEASURE, COMFORT, AND SURVIVAL

We eat, of course, in order to live. We eat to survive. We take pleasure in our eating because, quite simply, it is a pleasurable experience. Foods can taste good when prepared well. Sharing a meal with family, friends, and colleagues brings us pleasure, helps us bond over common appreciations of taste, smell, texture, and appearance. Eating food is a pleasurable experience. We also eat because our bodies crave to be fed, either out of hunger (it is time to eat because our bodies tell us it needs food), or out of habit (we gather for meals regularly whether or not we are hungry for a variety of reasons). Not only is food a comfort, but a meal can be a comfort of companionship and common pleasure. This is why eating alone just isn't as satisfying as eating with someone we love and appreciate.

For a person suffering from the disease of obesity, pleasure, comfort, and survival take on additional meaning with a lot of additional red-flag warnings. After struggling through endless diets, you may have learned that pleasure and comfort have to be sacrificed in order to survive. With KPP this is not the case. All three conditions must be balanced and addressed in order for the KPP protocols to have a lasting and life-changing effect. If eating is not pleasurable, you will not eat well. If you are struggling with hunger, you will not be comfortable. If you eat only in order to survive with no other considerations, feeling deprived of comfort and pleasure will not sustain the kind of change that is possible while curing the disease of obesity.

IS CHANGE POSSIBLE?

After years of following and surviving contradictory advice on what is the best way to address the disease of obesity, there comes a time when the honest person has to stop and ask himself/herself the question, "Is it possible for my situation to change?" Perhaps the more pressing question should be, "Am I willing and able to change in order for my situation to change?" It is easy to tell ourselves that we like new and exciting things, but down deep many of us simply want to move gently toward the unknown future that beckons. If we really wanted to change the circumstances of our life, we would look at how our life operates at the moment and do something very different.

Change comes at a price. If we change, those around us must change, or the situations in which we live and work, shift and change. Do we really want that to happen? In the case of the person who loses a considerable amount of weight, doesn't this set up a situation where other people are confronted by their own weight and, more so, perhaps their own unwillingness to address the obesity that they may be living with? If I tell myself that I am willing to make important changes in my life, am I also willing to assume the responsibility for helping those around me adjust to my changes? Change, as you can see, is a very slippery fish.

So, what constitutes change? Many people change only when confronted with trauma or a future that is impossible to imagine. Some change because they have hit rock bottom, and need to go in the opposite direction from the life they have been living, but is this really change, or is it merely accommodation? Do we really want to change our lives in order to live our lives? Can we embrace change as a constant factor in a life that is evolving toward new and healthier ways of living? Dare we change the way we think about ourselves so that we surprise ourselves when we discover the joys of living this exciting new way of life? Can we embrace the uncertainties that come with change in order to be the person we intuit we can become, perhaps for the first time in our life?

These are the kinds of questions that will undoubtedly come up if you start healing the disease of obesity with your physician's assistance. Your life will change. It will feel like new territory. Or perhaps it will feel like "original territory"—that is, the you that you've always known you could be. This simply requires willingness to embrace change on every level of your life. If you change one part of your life, you can change all of it.

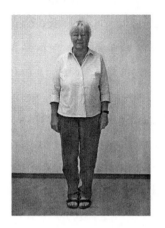

PATRICIA RINDY

Health Professional

I am a doctor of chiropractic and continue to carry my license as a registered nurse. I went back to school for chiropractic at age forty-two, and it was then that I realized I was old. During this time, I gained thirty pounds. Not only was I unable to lose this weight after graduation, but I continued gaining weight. I used to look at grossly overweight people and wonder how they could let themselves get to be that heavy. Unfortunately, I achieved a firsthand understanding of just how easy it was to get so heavy.

For years I tried various and assorted diet plans, but like so many before me, I found myself gaining all the weight back at a faster rate than I had lost it. Being a health professional, I certainly understood that it would be far better for me not to have lost at all than to rollercoaster with my weight. I finally told myself that I was getting on in years (at the ripe age of 57), and it didn't matter that I was so heavy, but it did matter. It mattered because it was painful for me to get down and play with my grandbabies. It mattered because I developed osteoarthritis in my joints and it was painful for me to ride in the car for any length of time. I have to drive an hour into work every day, and I was so ashamed to get out of the car at my office for fear that someone might notice how difficult it was for me. It mattered because my self-image was shattered. Shopping for clothes was a dismal experience and one I always dreaded. It mattered because my weight made shaving my legs difficult. It mattered because excess weight on a female my age predisposes people to cancer and, sure enough, four years ago I had to have a breast tumor removed. There were many reasons to lose weight, but what was I to do?

Then one day one of my patients waltzed into my office fifty pounds thinner than the last time I had seen her. She had been with me for eleven years and made many attempts to lose weight during that period of time. This attempt worked, and she was able to keep the weight off. She had been off the plan for at least three months, had not gained weight and had no desire to go back to her old eating habits. She told me that Dr. Kadile was one of the few doctors working with a hormone that actually resets your metabolism.

Well, I did a little research, and it did not take me long to give Dr. Kadile a call. I started with him in January, and was very impressed with the testing he did prior to beginning the program. Part I is all about preparing your body for the journey. Corrections were made in my problematic areas and by mid-March I was good to go. I have lost forty pounds. I am now on Part II and I know I am well on my way to losing the other forty pounds. The last time I saw Dr. Kadile, he commented on how my thyroid was decreasing in size. It had been enlarged for so long, I no longer noticed. What a thrill!

It has been the little things that have meant so much. I can now wrap myself in a normal-size bath towel with room to spare. I no longer have to stand in front of my closet in despair about what might fit. (I had long passed the stage of worrying about what looked good; I just wanted something that fit, as I could not bear to shop for yet another size up.) I've also noticed that my hot flashes have all but disappeared. Playing with my grandkids is once again a joy.

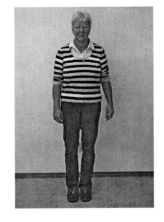

MOTIVATION IS EVERYTHING

That brings us to perhaps one of the most important questions that I or another KPP physician will ask you: WHY do you want to heal the disease of obesity? What is your motivation to take on the KPP protocols so that you can meet your goals? What drives you to get started and stay involved in the KadileAtric Power Principle® so that you can enjoy the success you've dedicated yourself to achieving?

Many of my patients start off wanting one thing at the beginning of the KPP protocols. Their goals and motivations may be simple and obvious: I want to feel better. I want to look better to my husband/wife. I want to see my toes again. I want to run a mile. I want to have sex again. I want to be proud of myself. I want to know that I can do this. I want to have energy for living, the joy of life again, and on and on. For my patients, they have achieved these goals and more. They have captured the energy and motivation of their desires and harnessed them to discipline. They have healed the disease of obesity and feel better and healthier in every way.

Then comes the next part. "What do I do with this life that I've managed to save?" For my patients, the new you needs to find new motivation, not only to stay healthy but to keep the weight off that you have worked so hard to lose. The motivation that brought you to KPP now shifts to living the new reality that you desired.

This is where I think the KPP program is unique: we not only help you lose weight and regain health but we help you transition to new and deeper levels of wellness because you will know more and more about how your body functions, what it needs, how it integrates with the life and lifestyle you want to live, and shape a new reality that you can enjoy, celebrate, and maintain. KPP patients must be willing to change and learn to change with enthusiasm and joy. As their motivations mature and change, so does the depth and degree of health they enjoy. Often, the new life is beyond anything my patients have imagined and enjoyed in the past.

So, you can see that the KadileAtric Power Principle® is not a diet. It is not about food (although food is an important part of the protocols). KPP is not a lose-weight plan that ends when the weight is lost. KPP is an ongoing, medically-supervised protocol to heal the disease of obesity that leads to a lifetime of new adventures in health and wellness. KPP requires a willingness to learn, or more specifically, to teach yourself about your life and health, your body, and how and why it functions. KPP is not a diet. It is an adventure in living.

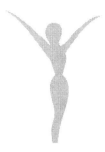

FOUR

THE KADILEATRIC POWER PRINCIPLE®—AN OVERVIEW

Most people do only what they are required to do,

but successful people do a little more.

—Anonymous

THE KADILEATRIC POWER PRINCIPLE®—AN OVERVIEW

So, now it's time for you to learn some of the components of the KadileAtric Power Principle®. Should you subscribe to the KPP program through your KPP medical provider, you will, of course, be given step-by-step, detailed instructions. You will know exactly what the doctor is doing and why he/she is doing it every time you visit the clinic. KPP staff will be available by phone or appointment to answer any of your questions or concerns about any aspect of the KPP program, and, as you progress in the KPP program, you will be changing your relationship to your doctor: from the doctor being an expert in healing the disease of obesity to being a trusted coach and colleague as you assume more and more responsibility for your ongoing care and well-being. By Part III (of four parts) of KPP the doctor will be putting you in the driver's seat and moving over to the passenger side of the car where he/she will help you navigate your way to your wellness goals, answer questions about the journey, alert you to dangers on the road, and congratulate you on the successes you have earned along the way.

Let's get started, shall we?

KPP PART I: PREPARATION

STAGE 1: DISCOVERY THROUGH "TESTING. TESTING."

You have probably attended a meeting at which someone gets up on the stage, taps a microphone gently, and whispers the words, "Testing. Testing." They do this, of course, in order to make sure that the microphone is working, that the sound levels are correct—not too loud, not too soft—all with the intent of ensuring that when the action begins, communication will be clear and direct. The message will be delivered and heard. That's exactly what happens in the first part of Part I of the KadileAtric Power Principle®. This is the stage of discovery through testing.

"WE'VE GOTTA TALK"

In the preliminary stage of Part I ("Preparation"), you will enjoy seemingly endless hours of personal attention from the KPP doctor and staff. They will ask you questions you may never have been asked by a doctor before. These questions will cover your entire medical history and that of your family. The questions will go into eating habits, sleeping habits, activity habits, medical conditions, good times and bad times, emotional patterns, and stress histories. This information is vitally important because it will uncover the underlying causes for your current medical condition. Since I believe that patients are not at fault for the disease of obesity from which they suffer, it is crucial that we have as deep and as broad an appreciation of your life experience as possible in order to demonstrate that there may be underlying causes that prevent you from being healthy at a healthy weight.

Together with your KPP medical provider, you will gradually come to see the patterns in your life and body that prevent you from losing weight and being healthy. Now, many physicians will ask a lot of questions when you first come to them, but let me assure you, few of them will ask the questions we will ask with as much breadth and depth of detail. Like detectives at a crime scene, we will search for the minutest detail of your experience. Often overlooked by most doctors, these can be the important clue to your being fit and healthy. The DISCOVERY stage sets the groundwork for everything that comes after.

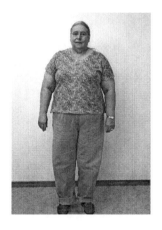

JOELENE KUROWSKI

I Looked Like Jabba the Hut

There is a picture of me; I looked like Jabba the Hut. I was so miserable in that picture. A young friend took that picture, and she put that picture as my Facebook page. I really hated it, and didn't know how to get it off of there, other than to put another picture on there that I figured would be just as bad. So, when I saw Dr. Kadile's ad, I thought "Well, maybe this could help." And it certainly has.

I had joint pain all over the place, and just didn't want to move, didn't want to go any place, didn't want to do anything. I was going to a chiropractor. I had to have my husband carry my laundry down to the basement so that I could do it. There were so many things I couldn't do and just so many things I didn't care to except to eat.

I'd gone to Weight Watchers several times and quit and tried doing other things by myself. Nothing seemed to work. This is the reason I decided that Dr. Kadile could help me. We have classic automobiles, which we take to car shows. My husband was taking the 1934 Plymouth to a car show and it started acting up. So, he pulled into a parking lot and we called AAA. I asked for somebody who knew how to deal with classic vehicles because I didn't want somebody who would wreck the vehicle. The fellow who came to help us just went on and on and on about how Dr. Kadile had saved his life because he had some kind of a situation where he had been at the emergency room so many times and they did all the wrong things, and he started going to Dr. Kadile. Dr. Kadile saved his life. He said that over and over and over again. So, when I saw the ad in the newspaper and recognized the name, and I thought well, if he saved his life, and he could get back on his feet and on that big tow vehicle, I betcha he could help me. When I had my first appointment with Dr. Kadile, he looked at me and said, "I'm going to put you back to the way God made you"—and he did. I now weigh 137. When I started I was 250.

Dr. Kadile would always tell me, "It's not your fault you're fat." It made sense because I would go to several doctors and they kept telling I had high blood pressure. It turns out that I don't. They were giving it to me because they—the women doctors anyway—the women doctors would all say, "Well, you've gotta lose weight and you've gotta take these pills and you have to … you have to … you have to …." So I just started studying up on pills they wanted me to take and reading about them and other medications. I found all kinds of negative stuff about medications, especially that they could make you gain weight and do all kinds of nasty things to your body.

What I find most of the time is that people think, "I'm not going to spend that money on a weight-loss program." It is expensive. Well, this is what I say to them. "I'm worth it." I have one son who just turned thirty-seven this month. He said, "Wow, Mom, your diet really works." He's seen me go up and down before, and my husband didn't think I could do it, and he's very proud.

You've gotta know you're worth it. Yeah, that's the way I feel—healthy!

One of the best things I can do now (that I wasn't able to do) is that I don't have to go into the handicapped bathroom in the restaurant. I can fit in the regular ones. I can walk right in and close the door. I can lift my own laundry basket. I can go for walks. I love walking because we live in the country—and looking at the trees especially in the fall when the leaves are so beautiful. My personality has changed. My mother has said that my whole personality has changed.

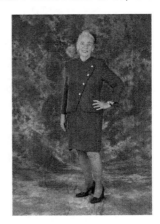

WEIGH EVERY DAY!

Even before the testing begins, I must insist that you immediately develop one very important habit: you must weigh yourself every day—yes, every day. You should do this immediately upon getting up in the morning after you've gone to the bathroom. Weigh yourself on a good, accurate scale, and record that weight. This simple habit is absolutely essential to your success in the KadileAtric Power Principle® program. It is the only way you will really know what your body is doing in response to the treatments you are about to undertake. An accurate and regular record of your weight is your best friend in this program. It is a habit that puts you in the driver's seat of your weight loss and recovery from the disease of obesity. Your body, through your weight, will tell you what foods work best for you and your health. Your scale will not lie to you, and will soon become your best friend, particularly when you start to lose weight, and KEEP IT OFF. I'm not kidding. Unless you are willing to pick up this simple habit of weighing every day, you will not have the reliable data you need to lose weight and maintain health. Your scale is your friend, one of the few who will be totally honest with you.

Once the interviews are underway, we will conduct a full battery of medical tests to determine scientifically what is going on in your body. Remember "Testing. Testing."? These tests will give us an "inside look" at how your body is functioning, how it takes in and utilizes nutrients, and how the various systems in your body are balanced and integrated with each other. Much like tuning up a car, we will study how the engine works, what fuels work best for this kind of engine, what contaminants might be reducing the efficiency of the engine, what support components of the engine are helping or hurting its efficiency, and so forth.

"THIS IS A TEST"

The medical tests will be conducted via blood, saliva, hair, urine, and stool samples. These tests include a comprehensive metabolic panel, fasting insulin, lipid panel, electrolytes, protein levels, uric acid levels, HbA1C, latent gout, liver, kidney and thyroid functions (including TSH and FTI), iodine levels, cortico-adrenal sufficiency, essential fatty acid panel, vitamin D3 levels, RAST IgE food allergy test, and a test for toxic metals exposure (RBMA/hair mineral toxicity). All of these tests and their exotic acronyms might seem a bit over the top to the average layperson, but they represent a range of testing and analysis far beyond the normal exploratory range of most doctors treating patients with the disease of obesity. They most certainly are not included in the over-the-counter diet programs that most obese people have tried and found frustrating and disappointing. The results of these tests will mean a great deal to your doctor, and as we put together the "puzzle pieces" of your medical situation.

These tests are at the heart of my "It's not your fault" philosophy of weight loss. Far too many times people force themselves to lose weight from a body that is not equipped to lose weight. In fact, many so-called diet and exercise programs actually work against weight loss, causing the obese person to work twice as hard for minimal results. This seems cruel to me, and I'm on a crusade to change the odds.

Once the underlying causes of weight gain have been identified, the human body will begin to heal itself, lose unnecessary weight, and begin to function again in the way it was designed by its Creator. The human body has enormous capacities to heal itself, but this capacity is unlocked only when the body has what it needs to heal and those factors that prevent it from healing have been removed. Bottom line: your body wants what you want—namely, health, balance, and freedom. Let's get on with this wonderful experience: you and your body as companions in healing and wellness.

Another aspect of the testing stage of Part I of KPP is to look at the foods you are eating and how your body handles them. Many foods that we commonly eat and crave are often found to be the foods we are allergic to. Yes, we often crave foods to which we are allergic because our bodies react to these foods with an initial sense of stimulation or satisfaction or comfort. If food is medicine, we tend to self-medicate through food, often choosing foods that give us a hit in the short run, and cause us to suffer in the long run. Not unlike an addiction to, say, alcohol or tobacco, people turn to them because of an initial "high" and then struggle to sustain that "high" by taking more of the substance that eventually hurts us. It is the same with food.

Some of the foods that many people are allergic to, foods that contribute to weight gain are: baker's yeast (breads), beef, pork, chicken, milk, corn, egg (whites and/or yolks), peanuts, soybeans, sugar, tomatoes, wheat, and white potatoes. Are some of these staples of your diet? Do you have trouble losing weight when you eat these foods? Are some of these foods your "comfort foods" to which you turn to make yourself feel better? If so, the second stage of Part I ("Preparation") of the KadileAtric Power Principle® protocols begins.

STAGE 2: REPAIR: PUTTING THE PIECES TOGETHER AND TAKING ACTION.

You are now ready to start using the information from the discovery stage of Part I and put it to work. All the answers to all questions you've been asked will be studied and a plan of action to get your body back in balance will be developed. Information leads to action. So, let's get started.

I call this stage of Part I "Repair and Replace: Putting the Pieces Together and Taking Action." This is a clear and accurate description of what happens. Your body begins to repair itself once it has been put back in natural balance either by adding natural medications and supplements that your body currently lacks in doses suited specifically to your testing profile, or by changing your diet to eliminate the foods that keep you from losing weight. Rebalancing will be the operative word here because our only goal in this phase is to "make a space" for your body to begin to heal itself and repair itself. The wisdom in your body begins to be unlocked from the vault created by the nutritional imbalances, invasive digestive forces, allergic factors, environmental challenges, genetic burdens, and the many other factors that have prevented your body from doing what it was designed to do—namely, heal itself. Your body is free to heal itself.

At this stage your KPP medical provider may prescribe natural forms of medications that supplement your current glandular and hormonal levels. The ultrasensitive testing done in Stage 1 of this KPP phase will determine where to begin, and throughout your KPP treatment these tests will be repeated to make sure that the optimal balances in these systems are achieved *and* maintained. Just as important as getting these tests is the requirement that you, the patient, know what the tests are looking for, what the numbers and ratios of the test results mean, and what the treatments are trying to achieve. You must and will be kept in the loop whenever you are part of a KPP program, because by the time you start Part IV of the KadileAtric Power Principle°, you and your doctor will be colleagues consulting together on your health and well-being.

STAGE 3: REPLACE: CHANGING THE FOODS YOU EAT

Food is medicine. This is a basic tenant of KPP. Good food equals good health. Good foods are those foods that your particular body can digest, incorporate into a full range of nutrients, and be used to heal the entire organism. Good foods are not highly refined foods. Good foods are organic with no synthetic or chemical agents used in the processing. Good foods do not contain environmental toxins. The outcome is overall wellness, but a remarkable side effect is, more often than not, weight loss that is surprisingly easy and effective.

Perhaps the most radical step many KPP patients will be making is replacing the highly processed foods in their pantry with whole, natural, minimally processed fresh food. For many people, food is that stuff that comes out of a box or a container. Inside that box (you can read it on the labels) is not only a food that was once originally fresh and good, but now, after suffering at the hands of processing machines, has been injected with chemicals and additives in order to keep the food from spoiling, to keep it looking good, or to give it a longer shelf life. Processed foods are full of things that easily contribute to weight gain and prevent weight loss. Highly processed food is not healthy food. It is a chemical soup, and the human body is not built for it.

Eating highly processed foods is also very counterproductive to the detoxification and cleansing that takes place in the testing part of Part I of the KadileAtric Power Principle® protocols. In order to get the body to rebalance, it shouldn't have to fight synthetic and chemical substances that cause the body to be out of balance. This is just common sense.

Also in this stage of Part I of KPP you may begin to make changes in your eating habits. Based on testing results and some good hard science, you will begin to take foods out of your pantry that prevent you from losing weight, while including foods in your diet that start to bring your body's natural cycles back in balance. Often, in just this first phase of KPP, patients start to lose weight that they never thought they could lose, and more often than not, without feeling hungry between meals. This is a very exciting part of the KPP protocols for my patients. They start to get results even before they start the rapid weight-loss part of the program. By changing some very basic eating habits, patients start to feel the difference in their body as it finds a new normal. Often, aches and pains disappear. Sometimes patients find that their regular physician will see signs of change with their ongoing medical treatments, often changing or removing medications for conditions that have improved or disappeared, simply by changing the types and amounts of foods they eat.

KPP protocols may also require that patients start taking natural vitamin and mineral supplements that enhance the effectiveness of the glandular and hormonal systems that are beginning to become balanced by prescription medications administered through the program. Each patient will have his or her own unique supplement protocol based on the extensive testing done in Part I and prescribed to offset any deficiencies encountered through changes in diet in Part I. These supplements must be of the highest quality and keenest purity and will be provided through your KPP provider clinic. The quality and purity must be high because the testing and treatment is done at a very refined level.

This focus on deep analysis of a patient's condition and bodily functioning requires treatment at the same level of refinement and purity. There is no such thing as a one-size-fits-all approach to a KPP protocol. Each patient's condition is studied and treated with precision care and individual attention. Throughout KPP treatment the patient's condition is monitored and adjusted as ongoing testing requires. Treatments change as conditions improve. Some supplements remain as staples. Some change, based on observation and analysis of the patient's condition. For these reasons, the doctor–patient relationship in KPP must be based on clear, accurate, and honest communication and trust. The doctor trusts the patient as the patient trusts the doctor. This foundation from the beginning will come to full fruition by Part IV.

Sometimes patients come from a toxic environment, either at home or at work, that prevents weight loss from occurring. Be they heavy metals or chemicals in the home or workplace, a patient's body will react to the toxicity by inflammation (a condition often undetected by a general physician), stress on other body systems and functions, or weight gain. Once these toxic elements are identified and addressed (through a variety of means) patients often start to lose weight and feel better. Often other chronic medical conditions respond and improve as well—all this can happen while the patient is still only at the Part I phase!

Finally, your KPP provider will review with you all the medications and supplements you are currently taking to determine if any of them produce side effects that prevent weight loss, or, as they often do, cause weight gain. Yes, the medications you take may be preventing you from losing weight. If this proves to be the case, your KPP provider will help you work with your regular medical provider to see if the medications you are taking are indeed necessary and to find substitutes that will address your medical condition but without the undesired side effects. This fragile balancing of good over better requires clear and honest communication among all physicians and the patient, creating a new team approach to the patient's medical well-being.

So, in summary, Part I of the KadileAtric Power Principle® is all about discovering how your body works, and getting it to work better. Through extensive and sophisticated testing as well as through a very thorough personal health inventory, your KPP provider will start to put together a detailed picture of how well or poorly your body is functioning. For those suffering from the disease of obesity, this may be the very first time so much attention has been given to the underlying causes of their condition. When this information is analyzed, a plan of action is developed to help the body repair itself by replacing negative factors with positive ones. Very often patients begin to lose weight almost effortlessly in Part I, simply because their bodies get what they need to do what they are designed to do: heal.

Today's preparation determines tomorrow's achievements.
—Dr. Robert Schuller

KPP PART II: ACCELERATED FAT-LOSS AND FIGURE TRANSFORMATION

Part II of the KadileAtric Power Principle® is almost like a dream come true. Perhaps in your wildest imagination you thought that it was possible to lose between one-half to a full pound in ONE DAY, and do this every day for several weeks at a time! If you dared to imagine this seemingly miraculous rapid weight loss, you probably assumed that it would take the willpower of a monk and include long days and nights of endless hunger. You may have already tried diets that professed quick weight loss, and they did, indeed, require enormous discipline and endurance, and on top of it all, you probably imagined doing this without a lot of energy to enjoy your success. If you've been watching those marathon diet reality programs on TV, you probably also expect to have to exercise until your tongue hangs out and you're ready to drop to the floor in surrender.

The difficulties and struggles of today are but the price we must pay for the accomplishments and victories of tomorrow.
—William J. H. Boetcker

Well, Part II of the KadileAtric Power Principle® is not like that at all. Yes, you will lose weight rapidly, and you will have to make some very conscious choices about when and what you eat, but you will not suffer endless days of hunger, and for many people the diet is so fascinating that they willingly make unusual choices regarding portion and mealtime in order to sustain the amazing results that they are seeing. On top of that, the excitement alone of losing weight so rapidly (especially for the hard-to-lose, obese patient who has gone to excruciating lengths to lose even a few pounds) makes Part II one of the most adventuresome experiences the obese patient can have. What's more, patients in Part II begin to feel energetic and surprisingly fit and vital. Who could ask for a better experience of rapid weight loss? Patients should not experience wrinkling of facial skin or "turkey neck" in this phase of the program. This is exactly what KPP patients report.

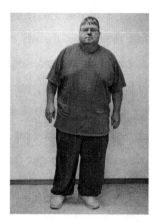

RICH JOHNSON

I Lost 160 Pounds

I needed to have surgery, and most of the doctors in the area would not touch me because of my weight. I knew that I was going to have to do something because the doctor who did my original surgery wouldn't touch me. He sent me to another doctor, and I was really excited because I was almost four hundred pounds, and I'd lost about twenty-five to thirty, and he also said, "I'm not going to touch you unless you lose another hundred!" I was shattered after losing twenty-five pounds. I thought I'd walk in and he'd say "Hey, Rich, let's go do the surgery," and after losing twenty-five or thirty pounds, I knew that losing a hundred would be next to impossible to do on my own.

I was actually recommended to Dr. Kadile by my wife's hairdresser. She'd had a good experience as well. Now, my wife does not like doctors.

She went in with me for my initial visit. Dr. Kadile looked at me and said things about my health that he could not possibly know. I didn't fill out any questionnaire or anything like that. My wife loved the fact that he could tell right away that I had serious thyroid problems. He just seemed to have an intuition as to what was going on with me before we even really talked to him. She really liked that, and when we left there, she said, "I really like that doctor. I love that doctor. He knows more about you than the guy you'd been seeing for five years."

It was pretty miserable because I needed a hip replacement. My quality of life was actually a zero. I had almost two and a half years of walkers, crutches, wheelchairs, and canes. My mobility was about 5 percent. I could get up and go to the bathroom, and that was about it, between the bad hip and everything else. I was always an active person. I played football and baseball in high school and college, semipro and everything. I had so many issues it was unbelievable.

Dr. Kadile's tag line, "It's not your fault you're fat," is so good. My friends would call me up and say, "It's not your fault you're fat" and hang up laughing. That's how they supported me. It means that there are so many underlying issues. It's very individualized, and I think people realize that very quickly when they're in his program.

It's really funny, when you go in and see Doc, you think he's going to talk to you and preach to you and tell you things, but I think he listens more, a lot more, than he talks. It seems like I say something and he could pull key issues out of what I tell him, right away, and I think personally that's what I like, because he was addressing my concerns and not other people's concerns, because, again, everybody's different.

And now my health situation is completely different. The amount of medications I was taking drastically came down. I had sleep apnea; I slept with a machine. I no longer sleep with a machine. I don't take regular blood pressure medication any more. I was borderline high cholesterol. I don't have that any more. My blood pressure's right on the money. These are very drastic changes. I think I was like the perfect storm for Doc. I haven't been heavy my whole life. It's been only in the last fifteen years or so that I got to be heavy. I think it just has to be time to do the right thing about my health, like the perfect storm. I had the doc on my side. I had to lose weight. I got tired of being sick, just tired of having one problem after another. Everything just fell into place for me at the right time, and it worked very well.

I had lost about 160 and gained about 20 of it back. A lot of it was semi-intentional, and as far as looking at me—you're not going to think I'm an amazing story or anything because I still weigh 240 pounds, but when you consider that I was almost 400 pounds...I've got spring in my step. I had a long time with walkers, wheelchairs, and crutches. My goal out of this was to have the surgery and get a few good years of life, and I've had that already, and so every day to me is just a bonus of feeling good.

And again, in general, you don't know how bad you feel because you don't know what it's like to feel good, and it's just weird. It's just amazing. Every day is just so great. As I said, all I was looking for was just a couple of good years, and I had those already, and I'm looking for several more now.

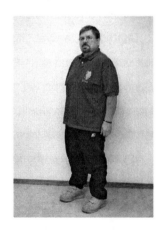

It's kind of like lotto. You can't win if you don't buy a ticket. If you don't take the first step, nothing's going to change.

Excessive exercise is prohibited during KPP Part II, because it is counterproductive. At a microcellular level, exercise creates triggers in the body that induce hunger. Exercise, in the KPP program, is recommended only after significant weight has been lost. Exercise is for the healthy body and not for the body struggling to come back into balance. We will encourage exercise in KPP as soon as it is obvious that your body is ready for it.

KPP Part II uses a restricted calorie, protein-rich diet with poly- and monounsaturated fats and low-glycemic carbohydrates to support rapid weight loss. This combination diet supports the metabolism in burning toxic fats that are deposited in the fat cells of the body rather than burning the supportive structural fats that are essential to health and healing. KPP patients will not necessarily count calories so much as weigh the foods they will eat in Part II. This is critical in order for the body to start burning fat reserve calories while getting the nutrients it needs.

THE INGREDIENT IN KPP PART II: RECOURSE HCG (HUMAN CHORIONIC GONADOTROPIN)

You couldn't be further from the truth if you were to think that the KadileAtric Power Principle® is just another hCG diet. Far from it. What I've done with the incredible research done on the effects of hCG in a controlled diet for weight loss is to incorporate hCG into a medically monitored program for optimal health, and on top of that I use by-prescription-only, pharmaceutical-grade hCG, not the easily purchased, over-the-counter homeopathic dosages that often do not produce long-lasting significant weight loss without hunger. hCG is an FDA-reviewed, prescription drug approved for the treatment of infertility. It can be prescribed by a licensed medical professional for other off-label uses.

So, What Is hCG, or Human Chorionic Gonadotropin? hCG is a substance produced in the body by both men and women, though women produce more of it. It is produced in fat cells, the liver and, most abundantly, in the placenta of pregnant women. This is where we find the biggest clue why hCG can help people lose weight. When a woman is pregnant and is producing healthy high levels of hCG, her body is capable of transferring fixed fat deposits back into the normal metabolic system where it can be drawn upon to make up for any nutritional deficit. This happens, of course, because the pregnant woman's body wants to provide maximum nutrition to the growing fetus and will now be able to use fat reserves to do so. hCG seems to be the mechanism that allows previously reserved and "unusable" fat to become energy and nutrition. In medical terminology it seems that hCG, produced in large quantities in the placenta, brings about a diencephalic (hypothalamus) change in the body.

Now, for the pregnant woman, the developing fetus is placing nutritional demands on the woman's body. The fetus requires additional nutrition and the hCG seems to be the factor that allows those nutrients to be drawn from reserved fat cells. For someone who is not pregnant, a very severe dietary restriction must take the place of the fetus for a limited duration of the KPP treatment, creating a nutritional "draw" that, with the presence of higher doses of hCG, causes a diencephalic change. Your body will start to use reserved "fat" for nutrition, a condition that was not possible prior to the hCG treatment. hCG also seems to create a food saturation level in the blood, which, in someone who is not pregnant, would account for why nonpregnant people do not usually feel hungry while taking hCG; their body is simply telling them that they are getting nutrients from stored reserves in the "fat" cells.

Physicians prescribing hCG usually deliver the drug by injection. KadileAtric Power Principle® protocols use a modified delivery system for convenience. We prefer a sublingual tablet, a small tablet placed under the tongue, held until it dissolves, and then swallowed. These tablets are taken only during Part II of KPP at the same time each day for the prescribed duration of the treatment (usually twenty-six or forty days depending on the patient's tolerance of the diet and ongoing weight loss without hunger). Women should start KPP Part II only after their menstrual period is over. They can continue hCG and dietary protocols while they are menstruating. On occasion some women will become extremely hungry for several days taking hCG during their period. Our protocols can be modified under medical supervision during this time and will not disrupt the rapid weight-loss effect.

THE KPP PART II PROTOCOLS

The KPP Part II protocols are very strict. They were first developed by Dr. T. W. Simeons, a British researcher, and have been refined over several decades of research and clinical practice. One course of hCG over either twenty-six or forty days can produce a weight loss of one half to one pound per day. For the obese patient who needs to lose more than thirty-four pounds, after a prescribed period of time, Part II hCG protocols may be repeated for a second or third course until the desired amount of weight has been lost.

Since we are using hCG to trick your body into turning reserved "fat" into usable nutrition, KPP protocols must be followed to the letter. Some of these protocols may even seem counterintuitive, but they are very important.

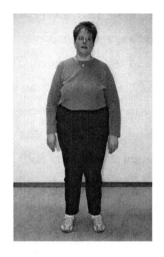

JANEEN OLSON

Easy Does It

Your KPP program has truly been life-changing for me. I have just begun my second round and am so excited to see more results. I am forty-four years old and never imagined I could have dramatic, quick results from any weight-loss program.

I have been overweight my entire life, and have lost and regained myself several times over the years. For me, weight loss has always been a struggle of calorie cutting and increased exercise. Sometimes I worked out for two to three hours a day, five or six days a week, to achieve a one- or two-pound loss for the week. Talk about frustration and struggling to keep motivated. I have never been closer than forty pounds to my weight goal and have often felt it was impossible to get there. So, of course, I return to eating poorly and not exercising, and guess what? The weight comes back, but after hearing about Dr. Kadile and getting involved in the program, those days are behind me, never to return.

The program is very easy to follow. Yes, Part II is restrictive, but if you follow it, you will not be hungry, and you will lose weight and inches. The best part about Part II is that it's short-term—twenty-six to forty days of restriction to lose the weight. I have never been on a diet with that time frame. It's usually hard to see any end in sight.

After losing the weight on Part II, and inches in the right places, I can wear clothes I wore when I was twenty pounds lighter. The program reshapes your body. It's amazing, and even a little weird some days, to watch the transformation, but seeing such quick and amazing results is a great motivator.

In fact, when I decided to do the program for twenty-six days, I wished I had decided to go longer because I was having such great success. The problem was I had events on my calendar and knew I'd be able to eat more variety in Part III. I would also have a chance to stabilize my weight before repeating Part II.

Part III was easy for me; I didn't regain any weight. Your weight will naturally fluctuate a pound or two, up or down, from day to day. In fact, some days, I went as low as three pounds below my final Part II weight. I love nuts and ate them freely on Part III, almost certain I'd gain some weight, but I never did. I even had movie popcorn. I just watched things closer the next day, and my weight was fine. The program really works the way it says it does. Believe me!

I am a busy attorney, wife, and mother. My five-year-old daughter is full of energy and deserves a mom who can run and play without complaining of aches and pains or being tired. Because of Dr. Kadile, I am on my way to being the best mom I can be.

My total weight loss was thirty pounds on Part I and II. On Part II, I lost five inches off my waist and five off my hips. My face is so much slimmer, and I can actually see my collarbone again.

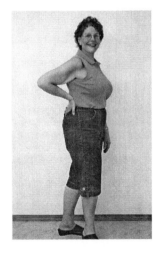

Here are the results of my last wellness screening: Total cholesterol dropped from 221 to 146; HDL went from 55 to 53; LDL plummeted from 140 to 74; triglycerides fell from 128 to 96; glucose decreased from 82 to 74. I can only imagine the continued improvement as I lose more weight.

KPP PART II: DAYS 1 AND 2

On Day 1, patients start taking their prescribed dose of my own compounded, pharmaceutical grade hCG, which I have developed under the name Recourse 2640. Recourse 2640 will be administered as a small pill placed under the tongue at the same time every day. It's easy, simple and effective.

The first two days of KPP Part II are high fat "loading" days. The purpose of this "loading" is to create fat reserves that can be used in the first three days of the restricted intake, or fasting, part of KPP Part II. You will be encouraged to eat as much as you want, particularly high-fat foods. Fat accumulated during these two days will not "stick" and will be used for energy. If you don't load up with fats these first two days, you will feel markedly hungrier during the subsequent calorie-restricted days. Many people think of pasta, ice cream, and bread when they think of fat, but these foods are carbohydrates. Fat comes from animal foods, so look for fatty animal cuts and prepare them with animal fat. These fatty foods include bacon, sausage, cheese, butter, fatty meats, and oily fish.

Some people might look at these two days as though they were a last meal before the gallows, but this is not the case. You will be able to eat your favorite foods again, but in moderation and with loving attention to what affect these foods have on your weight loss and weight maintenance. So, have fun in these two days. Use them as though they were an example of your doing something wonderful for your body, because by fattening up, you will ensure that your long-term weight loss will be successful and hunger free.

KPP PART II: DAYS 3 TO 26 (OR 40)

You will continue taking Recourse 2640 for the next twenty-four days (or thirty-eight days if you have been cleared for a forty-day course of hCG in Part II). You will also continue to weigh yourself as you have from the first day you started the KadileAtric Power Principle® protocols.

This is the part of the KPP that is most intriguing and exciting. Rapid weight loss! In order for Recourse 2640 to work, you must be on a calorie-restricted diet. This may feel like fasting but without hunger. In fact, most patients quickly start feeling renewed vigor and energy in this phase of KPP, a lightening and a sense of liveliness. When your body is in balance and starts using stored fat as nutrition, patients lose weight rapidly without the pangs of hunger or deprivation.

The diet must be very strict. You will be eating roughly 500 calories of food a day. This amount triggers your body (through the hCG effect) into using stored fat to get the additional calories needed for good health and well-being. You will be burning more than 500 calories a day, the additional calories (as many as 2,500) now released from the fat in your cells, nutrition that was previously not available for conversion to energy.

Recourse 2640 is believed to cause your hypothalamus to function and your metabolism to improve but only if you are not ingesting foods that do not interfere with the targeting of stored fat in the body. So, the diet will be fatty Slendergenic foods, high in protein, low in sugar and carbohydrates. You will be given a number of sample food plans and recipes during this part of KPP. The protocols you will be given will include the times you should eat, the kinds of foods you should eat and how to prepare them, as well as what to do when you go off the Slendergenic foods for a day by mistake or for a special reason. If you go off the Slendergenic foods for a day, or even just a meal during this critical time, you may be set back three days in weight loss and you will again be hungry. Your body won't lie to you, and if you trick it into deriving nutrition from stored fat, you must make sure that you are consistent and faithful.

The results, however, will be amazing. During this time, you will find yourself waking up in the morning, getting on your friend the scale, and reading eye-popping results. If you've had trouble losing weight in the past, imagine what it will be like to see your weight go down by a half-pound, a pound, possibly two or three pounds each day. This is exhilarating. You are losing weight while you sleep. You are not feeling hungry. You merely need to follow protocol, without excuses and without exception, during these very prescribed days of Recourse 2640 and Slendergenic foods. Pounds and inches are literally melting off your body. Your body is resculpting and reshaping.

KPP PART II: DAY 26 (OR DAY 40)

You will take your last pill twenty-six days after you've begun KPP Part II (or forty days depending on your physician's recommendation or disposition to remain on the restricted calorie Slendergenic foods). It is very important that you remain on the restricted Slendergenic foods for an additional three days after taking the last dose of Recourse 2640. These three extra days are an essential part of the treatment. If you start to eat "normally" when there is even a trace of Recourse 2610 in your body, you will put on weight at an alarming rate. It takes at least three days after stopping Recourse 2640 supplementation for your hCG to return to a normal level. Whether or not you continue Recourse 2640 for a longer course of forty days total, it is still very important to stay on the Slendergenic for three days after taking the last sublingual Recourse 2640 pill.

WHAT CAN I EAT IN KPP PART II?

This part of the KadileAtric Power Principle® is term limited. This is not how you will be expected to eat for the rest of your life, and the protocols are very simple, not a lot of choices. Just do it.

In summary:

- A minimum of 2 liters of water (10 glasses) a day, which may include tea or coffee
- 3.5 ounces of fatty protein twice a day
- 3.5 ounces of fresh vegetables (from a protocol-approved list) twice a day
- Two portions of a specified fruit per day, six hours apart
- No alcohol
- No dairy (milk, cheese, butter, except one tablespoon of milk per day)
- No oil (even in salad dressings), sugars, artificial sweeteners

EVERYTHING ELSE IS FORBIDDEN!

One thing that makes such Slendergenic foods doable, not just endurable, is that your enthusiasm and commitment is buoyed by the amazingly fast weight loss you will see each and every day. You will jump out of bed and run to the scale to see how much weight you've lost in just one day. You will be delighted with the results, and if, for one or two days, you don't see the results that you expect, I will be able to tell you why you might not be losing the pounds as expected and what to do about it. It's both that simple and that easy. Just follow the protocols and see the pounds roll off.

THE SLENDERGENIC MEAL PLAN

I've just told you, in a nutshell, what your diet will be like during KadileAtric Power Principle® Part II, and most importantly, I've told you why the Slendergenic foods are important. The foods you eat must help your body use the hCG to start burning previously unusable fatty deposits. Once you start KPP Part II, my medical staff will give you all the details you need to make the Slendergenic foods work for you and even become enjoyable. We have recipes and dozens of shopping and food-storage tips that allow you to maintain the strict regimen throughout this crucial part of the KPP program.

The Slendergenic meal plan is a special course of foods that help promote weight loss *for medical reasons*. This is done only after the protocols and testing of KPP Part I have discovered the underlying reasons why you have not been able to lose weight no matter how few calories you've taken and how much exercise you've done. In fact, you've discovered by now that there are "good" calories and "bad" food calories that control how your body metabolizes nutrients and stores unusable fat. You've also learned that exercise is very often counterproductive in the quest for losing weight.

The Slendergenic meal plan contains specific guidelines for choosing, measuring, and preparing foods. It is important to follow these protocols because they will keep you on target with your weight-loss goals while maintaining a consistent level of nutrition. Your body is going to use stored nutrition drawn from reserved fat cells, and you don't want to confuse this process by eating foods that the body would otherwise look for in your fat reserves. You will lose weight only if you follow these food protocols religiously during this critical rapid weight-loss phase of the KadileAtric Power Principle®.

FLUIDS

So, where do you start? Well, start with fluids, a minimum of two liters of water daily. That's the equivalent of one-half to one gallon of filtered or bottled water throughout the day. I encourage using filtered water over tap water because most tap water contains chlorine and fluoride, two chemicals that have been known to prevent weight loss. Black coffee (no creamer) and organic teas (in any quantity) can be included in your fluid-level goals. Do not use cream or cream substitutes (creamers) in your coffee. You may use up to one tablespoon of milk in your coffee per day. Under no circumstances should you use soda water, soda pop, or mineral water in your fluid-levels goals, and ABSOLUTELY no alcohol of any kind. Remember: alcohol metabolizes into sugars that prevent Recourse 2640 from going after the stored fat.

PROTEIN

Fatty animal proteins, preferably organic, are a vital part of the Slendergenic meal plan and they must be carefully measured. Twice daily you will be eating 3.5 ounces (before cooking) of fatty animal protein. This is roughly the size of a deck of cards, and it must be measured carefully on a food scale.

Oily fish, preferably wild-caught, is an ideal animal protein, especially when it is prepared with a minimal amount of fat and broiled, braised, or grilled. Most other kinds of seafood and shellfish are allowed as long as they are not farm-raised, pickled, dried, or smoked. Atlantic salmon is not recommended because it has been discovered to often contain contaminants.

Beef, venison, pork tenderloin, duck, chicken, and turkey (no skin, free-range is ideal), eggs, lamb, and veal are good animal protein choices, and, remember, they must be prepared with only a minimal amount of oil. Meats and fish should be organic if possible because nonorganic foods may contain hormones or antibiotics that can have a negative effect on your body when it is drawing nutrients from reserved fat.

VEGETABLES

Just as you have been rationed with animal protein, you are rationed with vegetables—only 3.5 ounces, twice a day. Your choices will be low-glycemic vegetables. You will be given a complete list of the dos and don'ts when it comes to vegetable choices, and you should adhere to these lists strictly. You may find that some of your favorite vegetables are FORBIDDEN during KPP Part II. I hope you can take these restrictions in stride, knowing that eating some of your favorite foods during this phase may slow or inhibit your healing and rapid weight loss. Some of these food restrictions will be only temporary. Some of your favorite foods may be returned to your diet in KPP Parts III and IV, but only after you have found your weight stabilizing and your health improving. Remember, KPP Part II is a critical and very restricted part of the entire four-part KPP protocol.

If you do things right at this time, you will find your dietary choices opening up in the future.

THE LITTLE EXTRAS

We have found that there are a number of "little extras" that can be used in KPP Part II to make eating enjoyable even while it is severely calorie-restricted. These tidbits include stevia as a sweetener, spices as seasonings, vinegars (except balsamic, which is too high in sugar), lemon juice, organic broths, and very small amounts of organic olive-oil cooking spray to help with protein preparation.

KADILEATRIC POWER PRINCIPLE® FOOD PYRAMID

PROTEINS:

Best Choice:

- Fresh white fish, halibut, haddock, bass, flounder, pike, brook trout, jewfish, John dory, snapper, sole, orange roughy, wild salmon, eel, tuna steaks, tuna canned in water, cod
- Crab meat, lobster, shrimp

Farm-raised fish, Atlantic salmon, dried, pickled, or smoked fish are not allowed.

Second-Best Choice:

- Beef
- Rabbit
- Venison

Third-Best Choice:

- Pork tenderloin

Fourth-Best Choice:

- Duck and goose, no skin

Last Choice:

- Chicken, no skin (free-range) and turkey
- Organic eggs, preferably only the egg white
- Lamb
- Veal
- Organ meats

CARBOHYDRATES:

- Low-glycemic

FATS AND OIL:

- Olive, extra virgin
- Butter
- Coconut, virgin
- Avocado

MEAL SUGGESTIONS:

- Breakfast: Begin your day with a medium-to-large breakfast consisting of protein (meats, eggs, cheese, or fish), vegetables and fruit.

- Snack: one apple and cheese
- Lunch: Large salad with a variety of vegetables and protein (from KPP Pyramid)
- Snack: Cottage cheese and fruit or deviled eggs and hummus
- Dinner: Large salad, steamed vegetables, and any variety of protein (from KPP Pyramid)
- Snack: 3 ounces of any variety of protein right before bedtime. This keeps your insulin under control through the night.

AVOID THE FOLLOWING:

- Avoid designer foods, which are foods found in boxes, jars, cans, and plastics;
- Refined sugars and any kind of sweetener including dextrose, sucrose, molasses, maple sugar, high-fructose corn syrup;
- Simple carbohydrates including flour products, cereals, breads, desserts, pastries, pastas, white rice, tortillas, chips, pretzels, and anything similar (zone pasta is allowed);
- Soft drinks and sodas—"bubbly" water like Perrier or Pellegrino is allowed;
- Fruit juice (high-glycemic);
- Bananas, grapes, figs, dates, and any dried fruit;
- High-glycemic vegetables such as potatoes, corn, yams, sweet potatoes. Also, be very careful with peas and carrots;
- Transfats, including hydrogenated or partially hydrogenated oils;
- Artificial sweeteners including aspartame, sucralose, NutraSweet, Splenda, saccharin;
- Monosodium glutamate (MSG);
- Nitrates, as in processed meats;
- Food from fast-food restaurants;
- Farm-raised fish.

LOTIONS AND CREAMS:

Body lotions and creams should be carefully chosen. Avoid these three ingredients:

- Mineral oil
- Propylene glycol
- Sodium laureth sulfate

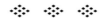

TESTING IS CRUCIAL IN KPP PART II TOO

It is extremely important to redo laboratory tests after KPP Part II to see whether abnormalities have been corrected appropriately and whether medications and nutritional supplements must be adjusted. Because your body is operating at a very high and sensitive nutritional level during KPP Part II, it is essential that we continue to perform our basic panel of tests to make sure that your body is operating like a fine-tuned machine. There are at least sixteen factors that I study when I order a metabolic panel of tests during KPP Part II. All of them have been monitored through KPP Part I, and now we need to make sure that the balance we worked to achieve in Part I is working effectively in Part II. This is why the KadileAtric Power Principle® isn't just a diet. It's a healing of the disease of obesity, based on real science, real medicine, and real results.

In summary, Part II of the KadileAtric Power Principle® ("Accelerated Fat-Loss and Figure Transformation") is the shortest of the four parts of the KPP program. It is the only part in which calories are restricted. This is also the part during which you will be rewarded every day for your efforts. In this part of the KPP program you can wake up every morning excited to step on the bathroom scale and scream, "I did it!" You might pinch yourself, wondering, "Is this real or am I dreaming?" You will see your body reshaping right before your eyes. Years of painful struggle with frustrating results are now a distant memory. Patients often cry with joy when they realize it was not their fault they were fat. Many patients had given up hope of losing weight and being free from the disease of obesity. Some patients had given up hope of ever enjoying shopping for clothes or of feeling healthy again. After this part of the program, they see that dreams can come true.

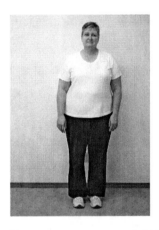

DEBRA ROWE

KPP Was Easy to Understand and Not as Difficult as I Feared.

I was having trouble controlling my weight. Everything that I was being told to do by every medical professional was not working. In fact, I kept going in the opposite direction, and both my primary physician and I were very concerned. At the time I didn't have any underlying medical health conditions such as diabetes, high blood pressure, high cholesterol, but it was going to be just a matter of time, given all this weight, before I developed those issues. That was my main motivation to see Dr. Kadile.

Well, it had gotten to the point where my weight was interfering with my lifestyle. I was trying to be active and exercise, but the exercise was ruining my knee joints. There were a lot of things I was giving up. I wasn't doing my cross-country skiing any more. My husband and I were talking about getting a sail boat to take on Lake Winnebago and, as I kept getting heavier and heavier, that wasn't going to be a reality. So we gave that up. There were things that I wanted to do that I couldn't do.

As I got quite a bit heavier, reaching a hundred pounds over what I should really be, it kind of seemed to me that people weren't treating me the same as other people. Sometimes I would be standing in line for services and it was as though people didn't even know that I was there. I'm a pretty large individual. How could you not see me? I tend to think that people were a lot less courteous to me. Oh, it wasn't really overt, just small things here and there, and I felt badly about that because I'm not that way to anyone else. I never have been.

Dr. Kadile was very clear about the program and that was so very encouraging to me because every time I would see him—well into the program—he would always say "It's not your fault. It's not your fault," and I understood what he was telling me: that at some point you have so much fat on your body that it just takes over, and it runs your body, and no matter what you do you just can't overcome the effects of the fat.

So, I started the program. I expected it to be much more difficult than it was for me. I just fully engaged with what Dr. Kadile was telling me, and as I got into the program, everything that he said would happen did happen. I started to have success right away just by bolstering my vitamin levels and changing a few things. I think potentially the hardest part was when I did the forty-day Part II as opposed to just the twenty-six-day of Part II. The forty-day was just a little long for me at that time. That's the rapid-weight-loss part, but I didn't find anything too difficult. What do you do? You do this, this, and this. You take these supplements. You eat these foods. You do that and the program works. I never felt deprived. If, for some reason, I would have felt deprived and had cravings like I always had before when trying other programs on my own, then that would have been difficult, but I didn't have that. I just followed the program.

For me, it wasn't that much of a radical lifestyle change. I know that for some people it would be, but I had already tried different things as far as my eating that were along similar lines, like focusing on the proteins. I already knew that starchy carbohydrates were not my friend. So I needed to give up on some of those things, and having to go gluten-free—because apparently I do have a bit of a sensitivity to that—was not that difficult because I had embraced eating more protein before I entered the program, and I had embraced being careful with starches already before I started the program. I didn't feel that—although there were changes that I needed to make—I didn't feel like it was a radical difference.

I saw it coming, and I wasn't distressed by it. I just needed to implement it more strictly and more carefully than I had before. Fortunately my children are grown and out of the home. So I didn't have to struggle with feeding the family, and my husband embraced what I was doing and for the most part ate the same kind of foods, and he just added extras. He could add the extra carbohydrates and the other foods that were not the best choices for me, and he's been satisfied. It wasn't an issue. So that made it easy for me as well.

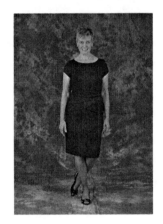

An error is not a mistake until you refuse to correct it.

—John F. Kennedy

KPP PART III: TRANSITION AND EXPERIENTIAL

Each part of the KadileAtric Power Principle®™ is a stepping stone on the path toward regaining full health. By the time you have completed KPP Part II, you are to be congratulated for the hard work and dedication you have shown in achieving you health goals and weight.

You are ready now to begin Part III of the KadileAtric Power Principle®. It is called "Transition and Experiential" for some very important reasons. KPP III will require you, the patient, to restructure your relationship with me or any other KPP provider. I say "restructure" because it has been my experience that most patients expect a doctor to tell them what to do about their health and they never move beyond that dynamic. Most patients just do what they're told and don't take the initiative to become more involved, take more responsibility for their ongoing health evaluation and treatments. In the KadileAtric Power Principle® you will not succeed if you stay in this rather immature relationship with me, your provider, or other KPP specialist. You must start doing your own evaluation, make your own adjustments, monitor your own habits, develop your own new goals for health and well-being, all the while you are learning how to maintain your new weight and health.

I cannot understate the importance of this part of the program, not only for your long-term health but also for your relationship with your KPP medical provider. You are embarking on a challenging new role with your doctor as you both navigate through this crucial phase of this new medical paradigm. This is another crucial difference between the KadileAtric Power Principle® and other weight-loss programs—notice that they don't address obesity as a disease, even if some of them actually use variants of hCG protocols.

As Bill Skaleski says, "It is very easy. There is no hype about it. It just works, and not only that, you are eating all the right stuff. No gimmicks, no things to drink or whatever. I have had to do some traveling, to attend some conventions and banquets. These places do not look favorably at a person on a diet. Free beer, free booze, and all kinds of food you should not eat. The diet is such that I have been able to take a few things along, just in case there was a meal I might have to totally pass on and grab a snack instead, but for the most part I have been able to live with these events and still follow the diet, because it is easy. There is a set of foods that are recommended and you look for those."

WHAT ARE WE TRANSITIONING FROM? WHAT ARE WE TRANSITIONING TO?

To put it succinctly: In KPP Part III you, the patient, are transitioning from being a compliant patient, to being an empowered, research-driven, self-care monitor. Up until this point your doctor has asked the questions, made the assessments, prescribed medicines, protocols, supplements, diets, and you, the patient (if motivated) has been a willing and compliant partner. Within this somewhat traditional physician–patient relationship, you have lost a significant amount of weight, feel terrific about your achievements, and honored your KPP provider as an expert and friend in helping do what you thought you could not do without help. Now you want to live the new healthy life that lies before you.

After having achieved many of your weight and health goals, the task you have before you is to take over from your KPP provider even more of the healing process. The role played by me or one of my KPP-trained medical providers (assisted by my expert staff) shifts toward being that of a teacher, coach, mentor, supporter, friend, and medical-research associate. We will continue to apply our medical expertise to monitor your evolving health and weight goals, but we will do so through your eyes with your lens on the camera. You are now the primary medical governor of your ongoing recovery and health.

This is a transition not only for you, the patient, but for your doctor—me—and my staff. We are used to patients who either comply or do not comply with our protocols. Now you, dear patient, have to begin our appointments with a different question: "Doctor, how can you help me learn the necessary behaviors and study my own medical condition so that I can take more responsibility for my healing and maintain my new weight?" In KPP Part III, I—we—shift gears. Together we will share the role of educator and co-researcher. You, the patient, are now the principle investigator and caregiver.

The essence of KPP Part III is the delicate and deliberate transfer of responsibility and authority for the patient's healing through education, personal research, and patient support. The patient is kept on track through ongoing monitoring of all the relevant physical systems involved in the first two parts of the KPP program. Now the patient will take more control of his or her success by learning why his or her body does what it does, and by conducting personal research into the foods, medicines, and environments that support ongoing healing. I and my staff, of course, will constantly assure the patient that he or she will always have a partner in healing in my clinic and staff.

Until now you were a passenger in the car being driven by your KPP physician and staff. In Part III you slide into the driver's seat and the physician goes to the passenger side of this healing vehicle.

Your KPP partners will be the copilots, giving direction, information, research techniques, ideas for adapting information to your healing needs and process and, yes, even recipes to prepare delicious and nutritious foods that help patients stay on the road to recovery.

Part III represents a critical turning point and challenge for both doctors and their patients struggling with the disease of obesity. The tools with which I and my KPP partners are most comfortable—analysis, diagnosis, prescription, and supervision of care and patient education—are gradually turned over to you, the patient. Encouraged to develop a growing attentiveness to your own health and eating habits, bodily reactions to foods, medicines, environment, and even social reactions, my patients start to learn to make important decisions. They learn to read the "signs of the road," monitor progress, check the meters, follow the map, all with my staff and care team supporting, encouraging, advising, coaching, caring, and directing their long-term recovery and healing.

By the time my patients enter KPP Part III, they should understand the basic concepts and medical protocols that guided me in making dramatic weight loss possible. You should, by now, understand the nature of the delicate balance that we sought to achieve, the way your body's systems interact, thrive, and recover. You should understand what I was looking for in Part I, and why it was important to follow the protocols in Part II. While this is a time for all of us to celebrate your success, it is also a time to shift gears and be in charge in a more dramatic way.

Patient education and support is key in KPP Part III. You, the patient, will be the primary regulator of the foods you eat, now understanding why and how the foods make a difference to health. The patient becomes a researcher into his or her own health and well-being. This is a very important part, because now you need to learn how to integrate normal eating routines. You must give your "new" body a chance to stabilize and establish a new weight set point. If you do not stabilize the weight lost in the first two parts, you will find yourself recapturing the weight. Now is the time for both of us, doctor and patient, to review what worked in KPP Parts I and II and why they were effective. It is imperative that you understand what was out of balance in Part I, why it might have been out of balance, and how it got back into balance. You must be fully aware of why the dietary changes in Part I were significant, and why they may have contributed to weight loss even before beginning Part II.

SO, WHAT REALLY HAPPENS IN KPP PART III?

When you've met your weight and health goals in KPP Parts I and II, in the KadileAtric Power Principle® Part III, you start to eat almost anything you want, up to what you perceive as being 80 percent satisfied—EXCEPT refined sugars and refined carbohydrates. This is the start of the transition process when patients learn to read their hunger and its satisfaction as a key indicator of how much food their body needs. If you feel stuffed, you have overeaten, and you will need to correct your portion size at your next meal.

After the strict weighing and counting of KPP Part II, KPP Part III will feel like entering the Promised Land of milk and honey. KPP Part II was a very long month (or month and a half) of weighing, measuring, portion controls, food selections, meal schedules, even though this month was filled with the excitement of losing weight rapidly. This is the time when my patients want to celebrate their success and endurance. They want to reward themselves, indulge themselves. Often patients will want to rush back to foods they have abandoned, disregarding the newfound self-knowledge that some of these foods are part of their food-allergy panel. Very often the foods people are addicted to are the refined sugars and carbohydrates that their body wasn't able to draw nutrition from. Patients often forget that if food is medicine, for them, not all food is good medicine. This is a time to celebrate, but it is also a dangerous time. It is a time when you, the patient, must take charge of the research into which foods in which quantities help you maintain the health and weight you struggled to achieve. You are now in the driver's seat, and I, your physician, am your coach, confidant, resident expert, and ongoing resource.

This is the time when my patients must become more and more informed as to what caused their weight gain and weight retention. They must know exactly why they suffered the disease of obesity and appreciate all of its underlying causes. My patients should become more and more curious as to how different foods cause them to gain weight, and which foods keep them at their new weight. They need to compensate or change medications that prevent them from maintaining their new weight, or look for sneaky environmental causes (toxic chemicals, metals, allergens, etc.) that triggered their bodies into states of silent inflammation, water retention, fat accumulation, metabolic "stalls," and all of the other underlying causes that created the disease of obesity they suffered. If it is true (and I profoundly believe that it is) that it's not your fault that you're fat, then you must be more than curious as to why you were fat in order to prevent yourself from becoming fat again.

My patients in KPP Part III know (because I and my staff stress it over and over again) that obesity is a symptom of a much more complex disease (or complex of diseases). They gained and held large amounts of weight because of a complex set of imbalances that included hormonal, glandular, dietary, social, cultural, and medicinal imbalances. Their obesity was not just weight-related, although their excess weight was the result and the cause of many of the other complex medical issues that were addressed in KPP Part I.

So, when you are set loose in KPP Part III to eat almost anything that you want (up to 80 percent of satiety), you must abide by the following restrictions:

- As in the first two KPP parts, you must weigh yourself every day. Without the scale to help you bear witness to your health and weight on a daily basis, you will "fudge," go by unreliable feelings and not hard evidence. You must resolve to weigh yourself every day for the rest of your life. Like flossing and brushing your teeth, weigh every day.
- Once you complete your course of the sublingual tablets of Recourse 2640, you must follow the Part II protocols for at least three days. This gives your body time to use up any residual hCG.
- On the fourth day after completing your course of Recourse 2640, you must increase your caloric intake by eating more protein and fat.
- Each meal should include *double* the amount of protein you consumed per meal in KPP Part II
- Each meal should include good omega-3 fats, as in extra virgin olive oil or organic coconut oil.
- You should not eat refined sugars or refined carbohydrates. These include flour or flour products such as cereals, breads, desserts, and pastas.

- You should not eat processed or "boxed" foods. You can simply ask yourself "Why would I want to make my body toxic all over again?"
- You deserve real food and real nutrition. Do not drink sodas, diet or regular. Eat foods that nature intended you to eat.
- Drink 8 to 16 ounces of chlorine/fluoride-free water (bottled or spring) before and after each meal.

This transition to a diet that works for your body is the central part of the KadileAtric Power Principle® Part III. You've learned what food allergies and sensitivities you have and what foods cause you other problems. By now you've learned if you are sodium sensitive, and if you wake up, weigh yourself, and find that you are a pound or a half-pound heavier, you will be prepared to think right away about what might have caused this small but significant weight gain. This is where you begin to teach yourself about yourself.

In KPP Part III my patients experience things that they may have never considered before, because they hadn't been informed about what a great role food plays in how they feel. It's not just about how good you look; it's about how much energy you have and what kind of quality of life you want to maintain.

Let's go back to my belief that food is often used as a drug. We must also notice (and record) how food effects our energy levels, our emotional vitality and our psychological well-being. If you wake up in the morning feeling sluggish, you need to check your food journal to see what you had for lunch the day before to identify the culprit. You must investigate how food affects your well-being and *take direct action* to address it. This is the perfect example of how you, dear patient, become the primary investigator in your own health-research project, and I and my staff are there as your clinical research support team to help you make it happen.

WHAT IF I START TO GAIN WEIGHT AGAIN?

In the KadileAtric Power Principle® protocols, we advise our patients to never allow themselves to gain more than two pounds. To keep track of this you must weigh every day. If you gain more than two pounds, you should fast for breakfast and lunch, and eat dinner before sunset. The digestive system slows down after sunset. Also, dinner should be either organic steak or wild-caught fish. You may have as many ounces as you need to satisfy yourself, along with an apple or a tomato. You can drink as much coffee, tea, or water as you like. When you weigh yourself in the morning you should see that those pounds are gone and you can resume your KPP Part III regimen again.

Human factors become the biggest issues during the patient-controlled practical aspects of KPP Part III. The patient is made to realize what makes him or her human. Human beings are hard-wired with unlimited longings and desires. We are more inclined to do bad things than good things. We create or invent what usually destroys us. Humans hate being told what to do; we learn well from failures or mistakes. Though there are no caloric or food restrictions, you may eat until you are 80 percent satisfied. Making these subjective choices and monitoring the direct results of these choices is a challenge many patients are both eager and reluctant to take on. My KPP staff will support you and continue to teach you to review the data you need to make good choices and enjoy the results that this empowerment can have in your life.

During KPP Part III ("Transition"), patients resume a typical three-square-meal habit. They can eat almost anything they want except for refined sugar, carbohydrates, and the foods that they have found cause them to gain weight. They should continue to follow the "law of 80 percent satisfaction." They can resume exercise, not to promote weight loss but to promote cardiopulmonary health and maintain muscle tone. They will continue hormonal supplementation and repeat lab tests as recommended and required. Most patients who are on prescription drugs are able to successfully reduce, modify, or discontinue them on the advice of their primary physician. Patients who wish or need to lose more weight after six to eight weeks on Part III can take another course of KPP Part II.

Failure is only postponed success as long as courage coaches ambition. The habit of persistence is the habit of victory.
—Herbert Kaufman

KPP PART IV: SUPERVISED DETOXIFICATION AND MORE SUBTLE LEVELS OF HEALING

It may seem rather odd to be reading this, but sometimes success can be its own worst enemy. Success can have drawbacks. By using the KadileAtric Power Principle® protocols, you feel better, look terrific, are knowledgeable about your health, know how to make good choices and, more often than not, make good healthy choices.

Herein lies the problem, however. You may have been feeling so bad for so long prior to KPP that this reprieve can prevent you from seeing that healing is ongoing, a continuum from good to optimum. You might feel better than you ever imagined feeling, but it is possible that there may be more healing, more well-being, and a more expansive experience of health yet in store for you. This is what I mean by more subtle levels of healing. Now that your weight and overall health have stabilized, we can work together to achieve a higher, subtler level of healing. If you have never known how good health can feel, you might equate health and well-being with merely being a hundred pounds lighter.

These subtle levels of healing are evidenced in better sleeping patterns, more vitality, increased concentration, a profound sense of wellness and well-being in the body and mind, fewer drops in daily energy levels, and improvement in interpersonal relationships because the physical distractions of subtle pain, anxiety, hunger, and craving, and so forth, have been eliminated or controlled. Now that the gross physical handicaps of the disease of obesity and its related diseases have been addressed, you are ready for the more subtle kinds of treatments that can make your life "zing."

The heart of achieving optimal health lies in (1) detoxification of pollutants within your body and environment, and (2) a realignment of your motivation for good health and improved well-being. Many wellness and well-being practices that you may have tried prior to KPP showed little or no benefit because your body and psyche were overcome by the power of excess weight and related diseases. Now, complementary wellness modalities such as massage, chiropractic, homeopathy and naturopathy, exercise and weight training, psychological counseling, life coaching, spiritual growth, and the hundreds of other healing paths that are available to us, can be far more effective than ever at taking you to the next level of healing.

All of this is possible because gross systemic imbalances have been addressed and a new norm has been established.

MOTIVATION: DO YOU NEED TO FIND A NEW MOTIVATION TO STAY HEALTHY?

When you first showed up at my KadileAtric Power Principle® office, aspects of your medical condition were obvious (excess weight), and your motivation was raw and acute. You were in pain, in fear, in doubt, in despair, and KPP offered you a path to health. Pain, fear, despair—these are powerful motivators, and ideally they kept you on course throughout the first three KPP parts.

In Part IV you must find new motivators to go further and deeper into the healing process. Let me give you some examples. I've had patients come to me with the primary motivation of not being embarrassed by their weight, or they wanted to be able to perform simple, everyday tasks without the chronic exhaustion that their weight caused them to suffer, or to recover their sex drive. One patient simply wanted to look better for her daughter's wedding. One might say, "Mission accomplished." In the first three KPP parts these motivators kept them compliant, disciplined, focused, and engaged. They were rewarded for their efforts. Now they want to celebrate the recovery of things they thought they had lost forever.

This is a good and a dangerous stage. Without real motivation, patients have been known to relapse, regain weight, reintroduce bad health and eating habits, and neglect the messages that they've learned to pay attention to in the previous months. They can get lazy and lose focus, or become undisciplined and nonattentive. They can backslide ever so slowly into a condition that they thought they would never ever be in again: overweight, unhappy, depressed, sick, and hopeless. It is at this point that a patient can become his or her own dream stealer, the one to take away the dream of a richer and fuller life experience in their body and mind. Without a realignment of motivation, patients can ever so subtly sabotage their evolving health and well-being.

At this stage, it is essential that you and I sit down and review absolutely everything you experienced during KPP and hope to experience in terms of the goal to be optimally healthy. You will need to pay particular attention to what might motivate you to chart a new course, learn new behaviors, and enjoy the new life you have worked so hard to bring about. You and I must not say, "Mission accomplished," until you have explored what kind of life you want beyond the weight loss, and how you hope to achieve it. If the gross motivators that brought you to address the disease of obesity are gone or hugely diminished (remember the power your weight had over your life?), you *must* find new motivators and establish new goals.

What are these motivators? Perhaps they are as simple as wanting to know more about what your body can do, what it is capable of. Perhaps, you want to feel good *every day*. Perhaps you no longer want health issues to get in the way of your relationships, your work, your spiritual growth, intellectual acuity, the contributions that you can now make to your community, society and the world. *New motivators for a new norm*, this is what is required.

DETOXIFICATION: "GETTING THE BUGS OUT"

KadileAtric Power Principle® Part IV ("Supervised Detoxification") is an extension and an enhancement of KadileAtric Power Principle® Part III ("Transition"). The major difference is that now, when your system is more in balance and weight is controlled and maintained, the effects of toxic substances from the environment will be both more profound and subtle. Together, now, we will turn our attention to the subtle effect that untreated toxicity can have on overall health and well-being. Detoxification is the key.

If your environment or job exposes you to toxic metals or chemicals, now is the time to be tested again for those toxins. If the results show high levels of toxic metals, we need to treat that condition by using chelation, the IV medical procedure that removes toxic metals. In order to maintain optimal weight and health, it is important that toxins are reduced to an allowable level.

The brain is the biggest fat organ in the body, and experts show that toxic metals are "fat lovers" and can seep into the brain. Some studies show that toxic metals can stimulate the feeding center in the brain. That's why, at the Center for Integrative Medicine, we've always said, "It's not your fault you're fat®." Hunger, cravings and overeating are a consequence, not the cause, of the disease of obesity. Depending on the level of toxins, chelation may need to be an ongoing procedure. Chelation should be performed only by a medically trained doctor who thoroughly understands its effectiveness and why it is used.

Up to 99.9 percent of people have chemicals in their blood. Just by playing golf, you can be exposed to all kinds of pesticides on the course. These pesticides are estrogenic compounds. The only known effective detoxification procedure for chemical problems is a low-heat, infrared sauna. These relatively inexpensive saunas can be purchased and stored at home. Low heat is optimal because it promotes the sweating of oil, instead of water, which is what high-heat saunas produce. Toxins are stored in body fat.

Low-heat saunas are available as single-person units that can easily be installed in a bedroom. Ideally, they should be installed inside the house, but they have to be specially built and require certification that they are environmentally approved. Patients should take a sauna at least once a week. They will notice the difference. They will feel good and clear-headed. The common report is, "Every time I get out of there, I feel clean, I can think better, I'm getting those toxins out of my brain."

FAMILY AND COMMUNITY SUPPORT: WE'RE ALL IN THIS TOGETHER

We may say we want our spouses and friends to be healthy and happy, but when a spouse or significant other really sees change happening, things can get very interesting. When one person in a closed and important social system changes, everyone finds that they have to change. You may need lots of support to navigate through the waters of change as you flow through your social network. This may be accomplished by teaching family and friends about the KPP protocols and their underlying science. This might also be accomplished by asking family members to sit in on some of your KPP clinic visits during this part of the program.

There is a human dynamic throughout the KadileAtric Power Principle® system. In the beginning it is very important to get family and friends on board, keep them informed, and help them understand what you will need, experience, and go through in KPP. It is important to keep your family and social circle on board, encourage them to talk about the experience of what you, their parent, colleague, or friend, is trying to do to heal the disease of obesity. Your family members may discover that they can enjoy foods that they either do not like or were not accustomed to seeing prepared in healthy ways. Some are probably grateful that they too got to enjoy eating fish and vegetables for the past few months.

Sometimes friends and family can become jealous and even sabotage a KPP patient's efforts. They may have thought that the program would be temporary and that they, as a system, could go back to the way things were. When you lose significant amounts of weight, you are bound to receive a lot of attention. It is imperative that you pay an equal amount of attention to your family network, members of which are experiencing changes of their own.

You have to make certain that your family and friends know that after all the hard work and dedication you put into your healing, you now are committed to keeping yourself healthy in the years ahead. You should remind your social network that unless you stick to the program, you could again face the agonies of joint pain, lack of energy and focus, depression, social ostracism, diabetes, heart disease, cardiopulmonary stress, and the many other afflictions that accompany the disease of obesity. Weight gain is an insidious process, and losing weight is pretty tough too. You didn't get healthy by yourself, nor should you be expected to stay healthy on your own.

Remember, there are many dream stealers out there. They come well disguised; they could be loved ones, relatives, or friends. Stay alert and find the support you need in this part of the process.

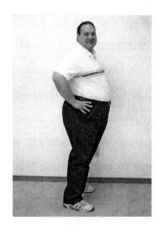

ANDREW J. TROFKA

A Family Affair

I was grossly overweight. My eating was out of control. I felt sick, and I thought I was dying. My blood pressure was high. My blood sugar was high from eating so many carbohydrates, and my cholesterol was high. Everything I had done in the past failed me. I could lose some weight, but I couldn't keep it off for very long. It kept going up and down. I had struggled with my weight most of my life, and in the 1990s I had gained more weight than ever. I was in the shower one morning getting ready for work and feeling at my worst. I prayed to God to help me. The answer to that prayer came a couple of weeks later when my sister Barb told me about my nephew Adam's success with weight loss and that he was seeing a doctor in Green Bay. She suggested that I make an appointment to see Dr. Kadile. Fortunately, I was able to get in and have some tests done in the middle of January before a vacation to Cancun for the wedding of my other nephew, Jason. I had my appointment and testing, and the follow-up was scheduled in February, after I got back. The "before" picture from Cancun pretty much tells it all. I looked horrible, and I felt even worse.

At the follow-up appointment, Dr. Kadile went over my tests and pointed out why I was so overweight, and the underlying causes. The most significant was my food allergies. I was allergic to eggs, peanuts, tomatoes, wheat, and soy, as well as the shellfish that I had known about for years. He assured me that he would be able to get me healthy with his plan. Within a few days, I started feeling better and the congestion in my head was gone. For years I took antihistamines and nasal sprays. No longer needed.

Within a month I had lost around twenty pounds and by April I had lost about thirty and was feeling better. In March my company sponsored a "Biggest Loser" contest. I entered as a solo contestant. I won the contest and was featured in the company newspaper. I was dropping weight quickly, and all my friends, coworkers, and family noticed it.

I've now lost over a hundred pounds and I feel great. Dr. Kadile can attest that my blood pressure is at normal levels, my cholesterol is perfect, and my blood sugar is normal. My regular doctor was pleased that, at my yearly physical, all of my tests came back normal and perfect.

I'm able to maintain my weight loss and have the tools to keep it off for good. Did I have some slip-ups? Sure, but with what Dr. Kadile taught me, I know how to get right back on track. I still have a few more pounds to lose, but that'll be a cinch. People ask me if it was really difficult to lose weight this way and I always respond with, "No, it was easy because I was willing to do what it took and followed the program to a T." You see, it really was up to me, and my mindset.

My family is a big part of my inspiration. My sister-in-law, brother, sister, niece, and nephew have all enjoyed success with the KPP. That helps keep me motivated. I'm so proud of them, especially my brother, Paul. We're very blessed that we met Dr. Kadile. From day one, he and his staff have always cared about us a great deal and coached us to be successful. It's made all the difference in my life, and it's done wonders for my family.

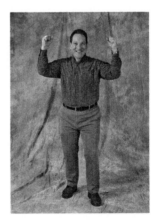

Success is a journey, not a destination.

—Ben Sweetland

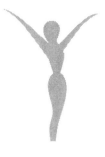

IN CONCLUSION: CAN WE HEAL THE DISEASE OF OBESITY?

Don't join the quitters of the world...doing what was

easy, rather than doing what was necessary.

—Anonymous

IN CONCLUSION: CAN WE HEAL THE DISEASE OF OBESITY?

More often than not, people begin to address the disease of obesity through the KadileAtric Power Principle® protocols when their "immortality" is challenged. A significant weight problem becomes something that can no longer be shrugged off when the consequences of ignoring it are life-threatening. Perhaps a patient's kidney function is impaired, or she has to take daily insulin shots. Perhaps a patient finds himself on a transplant or amputation list. Perhaps cardiopulmonary complications have robbed the patient of every activity he or she once found enjoyable and meaningful.

Striving for success without hard work is like trying
to harvest where you haven't planted.
—David Bly

By the time they visit our office, people are usually pretty desperate to address their disease and start KadileAtric Power Principle® protocols. They are exactly the type of people who commonly experience a two- or three-pound daily weight loss on the KPP protocols. After they lose a significant amount of weight, many need to start cutting back on their insulin. This sort of feedback tells me that the KPP system works. In our practice we have quite a few patients who, after losing weight, have been removed from heart and kidney transplant lists or escaped amputation of a limb.

Besides weight loss, other benefits of the KadileAtric Power Principle® system include a decrease in blood-sugar levels and blood pressure. Even during the first part of KPP Part II, patients often are able to reduce their prescription medications. Food allergies or asthma symptoms may improve. Some patients have gained relief from chronic sinus problems. Besides obesity, there are many other conditions that the KadileAtric Power Principle® protocols resolve. Once their weight-loss goals have been achieved, it is crucial that patients keep living the cure.

The KadileAtric Power Principle® protocols offer a dramatic resculpting of the body. The emotional and psychosocial transformations can be just as powerful. This is part of the comprehensive nature of the KPP system. We take a holistic approach to healing the disease of obesity. Everything changes. Many patients think they will never succeed in their battle against obesity and have resigned themselves to their current size. Once they enroll in KPP however, things will start to look a lot different, and their emotional landscape can change dramatically. When someone has lost 40, 50, 60, 70, or 225 pounds, like one of our patients, life becomes a heck of a lot more manageable and a whole lot sweeter.

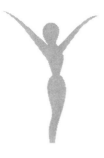

SIX

HOW MUCH DOES THE KADILEATRIC POWER PRINCIPLE® COST?

Whenever an individual or a business decides that success has been attained, progress stops.

—Thomas J. Watson

HOW MUCH DOES THE KADILEATRIC POWER PRINCIPLE® COST?

The KPP System, relatively speaking, is not inexpensive. It costs at least as much, if not more, than the leading diet programs that focus solely on the cosmetic aspects of weight, but it also costs considerably *less* than other diet and weight-loss programs that use in-patient, surgical, or psychological protocols.

Besides very expensive residential weight and diet rehabilitation programs, I know of no other medical treatment for the disease of obesity that is as comprehensive as the KadileAtric Power Principle®. This is solely because we look comprehensively at the whole patient and treat his or her condition as a disease, not as a moral or cosmetic issue. This is very important to consider when studying the cost of introducing KPP protocols to your life. KPP is effective because it does so much.

There is an interesting way to look at the math of a disease. Untreated, the disease of obesity is a very costly way to live (and live while feeling very unhealthy). The hidden costs, both to the individual and society, for not treating the obese patient are far greater than treating the disease.

- A 2009 study by the Centers for Disease Control and Prevention, along with RTI International, a nonprofit research group, found that the direct and indirect cost of obesity "is as high as $147 billion annually." The study was based on figures collected in 2006.

- The study found that in that year, obese patients spent an average of $1,429 more for their medical care than people within a normal weight range. That is a 42 percent higher cost for people who are obese.

Right now the mainstream medical community spends astronomical amounts of money to treat the individual consequences of obesity, such as heart disease, type-2 diabetes, arthritis, joint problems, and hip replacement. Likewise, it doesn't seem fair that health insurance companies pay to treat those conditions but may not necessarily pay for the medical care of weight loss.

While the KadileAtric Power Principle® System is an out-of-pocket expense, it is more affordable than gastric bypass surgery. Surgery can cost up to $34,000, and almost 20 percent of gastric bypass patients suffer complications that require follow-up surgery and additional costs.

ROBERT CARROLL

Is It Worth It?

So, do I think I got my money's worth? Absolutely! If I were to spend $100,000 on this program, I got $200,000 worth of health. I spent very, very much less than that—more around the price of a first-class, home-TV theater system. It is the best thing I've ever done in my entire life. Worth every penny of it.

But the only bad thing about the whole thing—a negative in the whole thing—is I had to buy a whole lot of new clothes. It's unbelievable, because I went from a forty-six-inch waist to a thirty-two-inch waist. Actually I was down to a thirty-inch, but then I got a little "fat," so now I'm back to a thirty-two-inch waist. Buying new clothes is the cheapest part of the whole program.

I lost so much weight that everybody thinks I've got cancer or something. We live in strange times when fat people are thought to be healthy and people who have lost weight are thought to be sick.

It's the best I've ever felt in over forty or fifty years. This is life-changing medicine, and that may be an understatement. I don't even know if it's strong enough. It's unbelievable. I feel like a porn star! I can only hope that other doctors and insurance companies will recognize this.

Insurance companies may cover some of the testing required through the KPP system. If you choose to start the KPP program, we will tell you exactly the costs you will have to bear and which costs might be covered by your insurance, such as medical tests and some treatment protocols.

When you subscribe to the KPP program, you are paying for one of the best medically monitored, weight-loss programs in the country. You are paying to receive the benefit of my years of in-depth research and successful clinical practice. You will be scheduled for eleven doctor visits throughout the course of your KPP I, II and III treatment, including a complete physical exam and an extensive initial consultation, and medical-grade testing throughout. If you know how much just one regular doctor visit costs, you can imagine the cost of eleven visits, and visits with KPP providers are usually much, much longer than the scant fifteen minutes given by many general medical providers. We never rush our patients through our office, and your appointments are scheduled to provide you as much time as you and the doctor need to keep your KPP treatment on course.

The real value of the KadileAtric Power Principle® is in discovering why it is not your fault that you haven't been able to lose weight, *and* in discovering how you can correct those underlying medical issues so that you can be free from the power of the weight that has been keeping your life buried under mountains of frustration, fatigue, disease, and hopelessness. Once my patients fully comprehend why they have not been able to be healed from the disease of obesity, they know that the price of their health is worth the freedom they now enjoy. The real value of the KPP program is priceless. You can have your health back, and weight loss is just the icing on the cake.

It may be less expensive for you to pay for healing than to be buried under the financial weight of your disease. Coverage and costs should not stop you from seeking treatment. Your health *and* well-being depend on it, and a life lived well is worth it. Your long-term health and well-being is priceless.

My patient Bill Skaleski said he was concerned about the cost of the program, but that his weight loss, plus success with his other medical problems, "helped me to overcome the obstacles of doubt that I had." Aside from the health improvements, he listed the top benefits he gained from KPP: "Number one has to be the tremendous increase in energy. Number two has to be the unbelievable self-confidence, self-respect, and pride that you feel in yourself again. You are no longer standing at the back of a group picture because you are fat.

"And then there's golf. My game was very bad and I was not playing that much, either, because it was very hard for me to play with that excess weight. As I began to lose the weight, I became more athletic and more athletic-looking. I was able to swing the club properly. I went from having some very questionable shots and trouble getting off the tee, to having over half of the longest drives in my golf league be mine.

"So, it has been a real pleasure to play golf again. As a matter of fact, I played seven times last week, and I do not think I played seven times all of last year!"

Finally, he said, "People come up to me now and they want to know what happened. How did it happen? They tell me that I really look great. They are reassured that I am not sick. I am just the opposite; I am feeling quite well, thank you!"

WHO IS ELEAZAR M. KADILE, MD?

It seems only fair that you take a look at my credentials as a physician when you evaluate the KadileAtric Power Principle®. I have a solid training and practice in traditional medicine, which I have augmented and expanded through ongoing medical education. I have mentored with outstanding medical doctors whose innovative research has become the foundation for my own growth and development as a medical professional. As I will report below, I moved into alternative, complementary, and integrative medicine to save the lives of my children and treat my aging father. I now take this motivation and experience to the service of all of my patients. The KadileAtric Power Principle® is the crowning achievement of my fifty years of medical training, research, and clinical practice.

As a graduate of the Cebu Institute of Medicine in Cebu City, Philippines, I started out practicing traditional medicine. I interned at St. Michael's Hospital in Milwaukee, and then spent my first year as a psychiatric resident at the Mental Health Institute in Independence, Iowa. My second and third years of residency were at Buffalo State Hospital in Buffalo, NY.

I am a diplomate of the American College for Advancement in Medicine. My memberships include: State Medical Society of Wisconsin, American College for Advancement in Medicine, American Academy of Environmental Medicine, American Board of Chelation Therapy, Association of American Physicians and

Surgeons, and International College of Integrative Medicine. I am also certified by the International Board of Environmental Medicine.

My shift toward alternative medicine began as a very personal journey about thirty years ago, when my son, Kristian, was diagnosed with systemic lupus, an autoimmune disease. Kristian was nine years old. Lupus is rare in someone so young, and the outcome is generally not good. The disease started to destroy his kidneys. Doctors could only offer high doses of medicine to suppress his immune system and the inflammation. Week after week my wife, Genia, and I witnessed the devastating effects of the drugs and the disease. Almost every month, Kristian was readmitted to the hospital with infections or drug reactions. This was the catalyst that forced me to seriously research and study complementary alternative medicine. We studied and traveled all over the country looking for answers, some of which worked, and some of which did not. Every aspect of our life was turned upside down in pursuit of complementary and alternative treatments for my son's condition.

As we implemented what we learned from the complementary alternative approaches, his lupus stabilized. He was able to resume his schooling and completed two years of college. Kristian opted for a kidney transplant, and I was his donor. The surgery was successful, but Kristian had a severe adverse reaction to the antirejection medication. He died. He was twenty-two years old.

Our daughter, Ann, was eight years old when signs of lupus developed as inflammation of her joints, especially her hands and fingers. The effect was not as severe as Kristian's because early on we applied the complementary alternative treatments that minimized the use of antirejection medications. Ann was in her third year of college when she underwent a kidney transplant. My wife was the donor and they both broke records for leaving the hospital very soon after surgery. I firmly believe that their quick recovery was the consequence of the science-based complementary approach that we applied. Ann went on to complete four years of college, is happily married, and leading a productive life.

In the early '80s my parents were living with Genia and me in this country. One morning, my eighty-nine-year-old father complained that his leg was heavy and getting bigger. I was shocked to see that his leg was blackened and almost gangrenous. I had an emergency consultation with a cardiologist. Studies were ordered, as well as a consultation with a vascular surgeon. The decision was to treat him with diuretics, and to wait and see. If he were not better in a month, he would need an amputation.

This was a devastating blow, not only to my father and to the family, but also to me, as his son and doctor. Coincidentally, at the time, I just completed a course in chelation therapy, a medical intravenous procedure using a chelating agent that binds and removes toxic metals from the body, but had not yet used it on anyone. My father's condition was getting worse; I had no choice but to make him my first chelation patient.

The IV procedure was done at my office, when no one was there. I watched my father anxiously for three hours as the chelating solution infused into his body. He awoke in the morning, complaining that he had urinated many times during the night. I looked at his leg; what I saw was beyond belief. The swelling had reduced significantly, the color had improved, and he said that it felt much lighter. We continued the chelation therapy for several months, and when he returned to the Philippines, he continued to receive the treatment from a local doctor, whom I trained. My father lived to be a hundred years old with both legs intact.

My father and daughter's experiences boosted my desire to pursue an alternative course, which, in turn, led to my current specialization.

Twenty-five years ago I became one of the pioneers in the emerging field of bariatric (weight-loss) medicine in the United States. Early on, I realized that dieters using conventional methods failed miserably because they were dealing with relentless physical hunger, cravings for sugar, salt and fat, uncontrollable urges to eat even when not hungry, poor metabolism, and an unusually high amount of stubborn fat in areas such as the hips, thighs, buttocks, and waist.

Unlike many of my colleagues, however, I wasn't satisfied with just dispensing drugs that never worked long-term. I set out on a twenty-year journey, traveling the globe and studying the clinical evidence behind nearly every weight-loss strategy out there.

I took the best of everything I studied and developed the comprehensive program I call the KadileAtric Power Principle®, an individualized, medically supervised method that reduces hunger, targets those troublesome fat-storage areas, rapidly burns the right fat, and resets the metabolism so patients can lose excess weight and keep it off.

I've been labeled a "contrarian," and sometimes several other less flattering names by some of the biggest names in government and the health establishment, but, hey, that's almost expected when you start questioning the status quo. What matters are the phenomenal results we achieve every day, helping people successfully lose weight. It has been unbelievably rewarding for me, more satisfying than anything else in my career.

ENDNOTES

1   Reinberg, S. "2010, Number of obese adults keeps rising, CDC says". *U.S.News & World Report, 1. Retrieved from http://search.proquest.com/docview/ 759646785?accountid=14872; http://www.usnews.com/articles/health-news/diet- fitness/2010/08/03/number-of-obese-adults-keeps-rising-cdc-says.html; http://www. usnews.com/articles/health-news/diet-fitness/2010/08/03/number-of-obese-adults- keeps-rising-cdc-says.html*

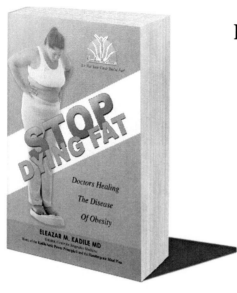

How can you use this book?

MOTIVATE

EDUCATE

THANK

INSPIRE

PROMOTE

CONNECT

Why have a custom version of *Stop Dying Fat?*

- Build personal bonds with customers, prospects, employees, donors, and key constituencies
- Develop a long-lasting reminder of your event, milestone, or celebration
- Provide a keepsake that inspires change in behavior and change in lives
- Deliver the ultimate "thank you" gift that remains on coffee tables and bookshelves
- Generate the "wow" factor

Books are thoughtful gifts that provide a genuine sentiment that other promotional items cannot express. They promote employee discussions and interaction, reinforce an event's meaning or location, and they make a lasting impression. Use your book to say "Thank You" and show people that you care.

CPSIA information can be obtained at www.ICGtesting.com
Printed in the USA
LVOW101003030613

336655LV00015B/382/P